The Future of Psychiatry as a Medical Specialty

ISSUES IN
PSYCHIATRY

Joseph Bloom, M.D.
Series Editor

The Future of Psychiatry
as a Medical Specialty

Joel Yager, M.D.

Professor, Department of Psychiatry and Biobehavioral Sciences, University of California at Los Angeles; Director of Residency Education, UCLA Neuropsychiatric Institute and West Los Angeles VA Medical Center (Brentwood Division); and Associate Chief of Staff for Residency Education, West Los Angeles VA Medical Center (Brentwood Division), Los Angeles, California

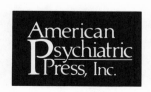

1400 K Street, N.W.
Washington, D.C. 20005

Copyright © 1989 American Psychiatric Press, Inc.
ALL RIGHTS RESERVED
Manufactured in the United States of America
89 90 91 92 4 3 2 1
First Edition

The paper used in this publication meets the minimum requirements of American National Standard for Information Sciences—Permanence of Paper for Printed Library Materials, ANSI Z39.48-1984.   ∞

Library of Congress Cataloging-in-Publication Data
The Future of psychiatry as a medical
      specialty.
      (Issues in psychiatry)
      Includes bibliographies.
      1. Psychiatry—Forecasting.   I. Yager, Joel.
II. Series. [DNLM: 1. Psychiatry—trends.
WM 21 F996]
RC455.2.F67F87   1989   616.89   88-34967
ISBN 0-88048-309-1 (alk. paper)

Contents

Contributors

Philip G. Bashook, Ed.D.
Director of Education
American Psychiatric Association

Adjunct Associate Professor of Psychiatry and Behavioral
  Science
George Washington University
Washington, D.C.

Jonathan F. Borus, M.D.
Associate Professor of Psychiatry
Harvard Medical School
Cambridge, Massachusetts

Director of Residency and Fellowship Training
Massachusetts General Hospital
Boston, Massachusetts

Marc Galanter, M.D.
Professor of Psychiatry
New York University

Director, Division of Alcoholism and Drug Abuse
New York University School of Medicine
New York, New York

Jeffrey L. Houpt, M.D.
Professor and Chairman
Department of Psychiatry
Emory University

Deputy Dean
Emory University School of Medicine
Atlanta, Georgia

Jerald Kay, M.D.
Professor of Child Psychiatry
University of Cincinnati College of Medicine

Director of Residency Training
Department of Psychiatry
University of Cincinnati School of Medicine
Cincinnati, Ohio

Donald G. Langsley, M.D.
Professor of Psychiatry and Behavioral Sciences
Northwestern University Medical School
Evanston, Illinois

Gayle E. Strauss, Ed.D.
Staff Research Associate
Department of Psychiatry and Biobehavioral Sciences
University of California at Los Angeles
Los Angeles, California

Gordon Strauss, M.D.
Associate Clinical Professor of Psychiatry
University of California at Los Angeles

Associate Director of Residency Education
University of California at Los Angeles Neuropsychiatric
    Institute
West Los Angeles VA Medical Center (Brentwood Division)
Los Angeles, California

Zebulon Taintor, M.D.
Professor and Vice Chairman of Psychiatry
New York University Medical Center

Chief of Staff
Manhattan Psychiatric Center
New York, New York

Past Assistant Director for Cost Considerations
National Institute of Mental Health
Rockville, Maryland

Allan Tasman, M.D.
Professor of Psychiatry
University of Connecticut Medical School

Director of Residency Training and Medical Student Education
Department of Psychiatry
University of Connecticut Medical School
Hartford, Connecticut

Sidney H. Weissman, M.D.
Director of Training and Education
Department of Psychiatry
Michael Reese Hospital and Medical Center

Associate Professor of Psychiatry
University of Chicago
Chicago, Illinois

Joel Yager, M.D.
Professor, Department of Psychiatry and Biobehavioral
    Sciences
University of California at Los Angeles

Director of Residency Education
University of California at Los Angeles Neuropsychiatric
    Institute/West Los Angeles VA Medical Center (Brentwood
    Division)

Associate Chief of Staff for Residency Education
West Los Angeles VA Medical Center (Brentwood Division)
Los Angeles, California

Preface

This book presents the collected views of a group of prominent psychiatric educators about the current state and likely future of psychiatry as a medical specialty. Such risky crystal-ball gazing is necessary for educators who must prepare today's and tomorrow's students for the profession they are likely to encounter in the future. The views represented are, of course, the best guesses of the authors, and may bear little or no resemblance to how psychiatry will actually appear in years to come. And, as befits a field as diverse as psychiatry, we are reassured by the fact that there is no unanimity of viewpoint, regarding either what psychiatry is likely to be or what psychiatry should be like, set forth.

We start with a rough estimate of what psychiatry currently is. In Chapter 1, Donald G. Langsley and I describe the evolution of contemporary psychiatry through several ideological and practice revolutions, and then consider the present outlines of the profession as operationally defined by the skills and knowledge that a large percentage of academic and practicing psychiatrists agree should be within the domain of the general psychiatrist at this point in the profession's history.

In Chapter 2, Jonathan F. Borus considers the influence that changes in practice settings and the economic forces besetting all of medicine are likely to have on the practice of psychiatry. The possibly profound impact of these forces must inform the profession as it struggles to decide how many and what types of psychiatrists to produce to meet future needs and demands; it must also inform today's trainees about the types of professional lives they can expect in the future.

Chapters 3 and 4, by Sidney H. Weissman and Philip G. Bashook and by me, struggle with the issue of subspecialization in psychiatry. In Chapter 3, Weissman and Bashook argue that we need to assure that the training of general psychiatrists continues, and that all psychiatrists, using a broad biopsychosocial perspective, remain well grounded and able to care for a diverse assortment of clinical problems. In Chapter 4, I describe what I believe to be inevitable trends toward subspecialization and offer some ways in which the profession and individuals can cope with these pressures.

Following the discussion of subspecialization, it is only fitting to consider some specifics, and Chapters 5 and 6 provide case examples. Jeffrey Houpt imagines the future of what in the past has been called consultation–liaison psychiatry and predicts, pending the suggestion of an alternative term, the emergence of *psychiatric medicine*. The highly specialized, often doubly trained and boarded psychiatrist–internist (or psychiatrist–pediatrician, etc.) may increasingly care for patients with complex and combined medical and psychiatric problems. Even within consultation psychiatry circles, this view has generated debate. The next area of emerging subspecialization considered is *addiction medicine*, ably discussed in Chapter 6 by Marc Galanter and Zebulon Taintor. They review current developments in the formation of fellowship programs and specialty societies and set forth specific educational programs for this frequently neglected area of psychiatric concern.

The future of psychiatric education at the medical student and residency-training level, at the heart of our concerns, is considered in Chapter 7 by Jerald Kay and Alan Tasman. They consider both curriculum and the impact that new teaching methods based on emerging technologies are likely to have on training programs.

In Chapter 8, Gordon and Gayle Strauss and I present additional data from a survey of a large number of psychiatric experts representing diverse areas of psychiatry. We conducted, earlier in the decade, a study we refer to as the "cutting edge." This study asked the experts to describe the major advances that had occurred in their respective fields in the past decade, and to predict the advances they believed most probable for the next.

Reviewing and critically commenting on all the preceding material, Zebulon Taintor, in Chapter 9, brings to bear his keen abilities at discernment by viewing psychiatry up to the present and into the future from both linear and cyclic perspectives of historical analysis. He takes well-reasoned issue with a number of observations and predictions offered in earlier chapters, adding to the vitality of the debates.

Finally, I present an overview of futuristic research with special reference to psychiatry in Chapter 10. I describe the major predictive methods of futurists and some of the most prominent predictions of the most prominent futurists for the world at large in the last half of the century that would impact psychiatry, and I review the predictions of psychiatry's own futurists. The chapter concludes with a few predictions of my own.

While it is hard to see exactly where the profession may go, readers can take some reassurance from the fact that all the authors concur that psychiatry WILL have a future, and that regardless of the many transformations that may occur in the process, it will very likely remain vigorous and energetic.

Joel Yager, M.D.

Chapter 1

What Is a Psychiatrist?

Donald G. Langsley, M.D.
Joel Yager, M.D.

The Revolutions in Psychiatry

Many attempts have been made to define *psychiatrists*, but the field keeps changing. In the past century, we have seen at least four psychiatric revolutions. In each revolution, the psychiatrist was redefined and the next hundred years promise more change. The 19th century saw psychiatry move from an era of custody and asylums to a period of humane care and an approach called *moral treatment*. Moral treatment wasn't treatment in today's sense, but rather a humanitarian type of custody for those who had previously been chained, reviled, and cast out from society, in much the same fashion as had the leper. Around the turn of the century, a second revolution was initiated with the psychology of Freud. It focused on concepts of determinism, unconscious forces in behavior, and hopes for a causal explanation of mental disorder, and treatment was directed at those factors presumed to be causative. Exciting developments in the concept of disease, knowledge of human physiology and pathophysiology abounded during this era. Scientific medicine began its remarkable advance in the 20th century and promised understanding of etiologies and hope for effective treatment. Psychiatric treatment expanded in the 1920s and 1930s, as empirical evidence that certain somatic treatments could improve the symptoms of the serious disorders was compiled. Psychotic patients improved, at least temporarily, when treated with chemicals (camphor, and later metrazole) that induced grand mal seizures. Chemical treatments gave way to electrical stimulation, a more controllable approach to inducing a convulsion. During the same era, insulin-induced hypoglycemic coma joined the somatic armamentarium of the psychiatrist, and not long afterward, surgical procedures on the brain itself (lobotomy, leucotomy) were in vogue, albeit temporarily. The influence of these empirical sciences was reflected in separation of psychiatrists into two major groups— the APs and DOs. The APs were analytical psychotherapy-oriented psychiatrists; they practiced in private offices and their patients manifested inhibitions, failure to achieve their full potential, and symptom neuroses or neurotic character traits. The DOs were directive-organically oriented psychiatrists, practicing in psychiatric hospitals and using predominantly somatic treatments. Their patients were the schizophrenics, manic-depressives, and those suffering from organic brain disorders. The psychiatrists of that era could be defined by their professional skills and activities.

The third psychiatric revolution was a product of the 1950s and 1960s. It included the development of community treatment, attention to the needs of whole populations, a move out of the state mental hospital (deinstitutionalization) to limited use of psychiatric wards in community general hospitals, a focus on the involvement of the family and other social therapies, and a hope that major mental disorders could truly be prevented or at least identified early enough to institute early intervention. Many feel that development of psychoactive medications had more influence than any other factor in developing treatment in the community, as the early 1950s saw the discovery that certain medications tranquilized disturbed patients and influenced psychotic symptoms. Antipsychotic drugs were soon followed by antidepressants and antianxiety drugs. Lithium, to prevent attacks of mania, became the major psychopharmacological breakthrough in prevention. Nonhospital treatment was made possible by a combination of medication and early psychotherapeutic intervention with patients and their families. During this period, crisis intervention became widely available, and it was shown that patients formerly in need of immediate hospitalization could be treated in the community by family crisis therapy. In that era of social reform, efforts to solve problems of poverty and racism set the stage for the hope that treatment of a community's ills would be reflected by improvement of the lot of the mentally disordered. Payment for the treatment of general illness by third parties (government and insurance plans) introduced coverage for psychiatric disorders, and it was tempting to define psychiatric patients as *ill* or as *patients*, rather than as the victims of social upheaval. The availability of payment for treatment in the community, as well as the discoveries of effective short-term treatments helped advance the cause of community psychiatry (the third psychiatric revolution); it also helped move the model from social and community cause and treatment to a scientific biomedical model.

The fourth psychiatric revolution has been a product of the 1970s and 1980s and doubtlessly will occupy at least the rest of this century. It arises from exciting new discoveries in biological sciences. The breakthroughs and promises of new information on the biology of psychosis and the genetics of major mental disorder and a better understanding of psychopharmacology will base psychiatric practice more heavily on biologically oriented sciences, and give it the biomedical underpinning common to other medical specialties. New discoveries do not require abandonment of the tried and true, and individual psychotherapy and the social therapies are not being abandoned in this fourth psychiatric revolution, but they will not constitute so large and exclusive a portion of psychiatric practice.

The current revolution is also being shaped by a number of social and economic forces. Among the strongest of these forces are current public and professional dissatisfactions with lifetime licensure and irrevocable certification for psychiatrists and all medical specialists. The public and the professions are taking note of a number of factors, which will be mentioned in detail in the sections that follow.

Malpractice Suits and Award Sizes

Whether one blames the legal profession or the medical profession, the fact is that malpractice has called the general skill of physicians into question. There is an implicit assumption that notorious malpractice suits and multimillion dollar awards are a consequence of physician incompetence. That incompetence is in part presumed to result from failure to maintain and update the skills acquired during medical school and graduate medical education.

Malpractice is a threat to all specialties. The costs of malpractice insurance have skyrocketed, and those costs have caused some specialists to give up their practices or some aspects of them. And, although the costs of insurance for psychiatrists do not approach those of obstetricians or neurosurgeons, they have quadrupled over the past three years. The fiscal implications are clear, but malpractice threats have also influenced psychiatric practice. To protect themselves against malpractice judgments, or even against just suits, many psychiatrists have become more cautious and are practicing *defensive* medicine. They have become more concerned about national standards and about using the most widely accepted treatment techniques. Some psychiatrists are refusing to treat the more litigious or complicated patients, and they are more inclined to use hospitalization. The high visibility of malpractice suits and the growing number of reports of suits for sexual involvement with patients has concerned the profession. In addition to the malpractice consequences of such behavior, the American Psychiatric Association (APA) has widely publicized its standards of ethics and has been especially vigorous in investigation of complaints about ethical and professional behaviors. The public has been subjected to a barrage of media reports about physician fraud and unethical behavior, lending further motivation to the need to adhere to high standards of practice. In fact, the federal government has now established a national Disciplinary Data Bank under Public Law 99-660. Under contract with the Department of Health and Human Services, this organization collects information about suspensions and revocations under state licensure acts, about malpractice judgments and settlements, and about changes in hospital medical staff membership or privileges. In the past, individual state licensure determinations allowed physicians to move from one state to another with relative ease, in the event of adverse action by a licensing board. Today's data banks and communication with the Federation of State Medical Boards (FSMB) or the American Medical Association (AMA) make it more difficult to establish practice in a new state when there has been licensure revocation or suspension.

Media Attention to Physician Disciplinary Activities

Licensure boards and government Medicare payers are increasing the frequency of their disciplinary actions toward physicians who commit fraud or who are practicing poor quality medicine. Some deficiencies constitute outright fraud, as when billing for services not rendered or considered medically unnecessary occurs. Others encompass unethical behavior toward patients in various forms, including sexual activity. The numbers of licensing board suspensions or revocations have increased visibly over the past five years, and better exchange of information through the Disciplinary Data Bank has heightened awareness. In an age of high media exposure, these events influence the perception of the medical profession.

Professional Review Organizations

These organizations, called PROs, initially focused on cost containment and utilization reviews. They have the authority to review medical care in hospital settings and are now moving into the ambulatory and office settings. These organizations are now shifting attention to quality assessment, and there have been recent reports of physicians in rural areas being denied Medicare reimbursement because of low quality care, i.e., failure to adhere to national standards.

Reregistration of Medical Licensure

Reregistration of medical licensure used to be a routine event requiring only the payment of a fee. Media notoriety and grand jury criticisms in New York State have resulted in a proposal for competence determination every nine years as a condition of reregistration of the license to practice medicine. Such a law already exists in Michigan, but it has yet to be enforced, in part because the methodology is not secure, but such proposals will doubtlessly extend to many, if not most states. Competence will probably be determined on the basis of performance assessments, with the evaluation of hospital practice based on record reviews and departmental plus committee reviews. The assessment for office-based practice will probably require a test of skills, plus an office record review.

Plans for Outcome Studies

The Joint Commission on Accreditation of Health Care Organizations (JCAH) is changing its focus from looking at structure to determine the quality of care to one involving process and outcome at an institutional level. The American Board of Medical Specialties (ABMS), the parent organization of the 23 specialty boards, has been interested in physician performance assessment as one technique for specialty recertification. It is natural for the ABMS and the Joint Commission on Accreditation of Health Care Organizations to combine efforts to develop techniques of physician performance assessment that can be applied to determining the quality of institutional care, as each institution is largely the sum of the work of its medical staff.

Recertification

All of the above factors have spurred the specialty certifying boards to move more rapidly into mandatory recertification. Recertification is important because the definition of a psychiatrist changes with discoveries in science and new methods of practice.

The need to maintain the medical knowledge and skill level of the specialist has been readily acknowledged since specialty certification developed in the 1930s. Proposals for periodic assessment of physician competence were advanced at the very time that the specialty boards were being organized and, in 1969, the American Board of Family Practice set a historic example by deciding to issue only time-limited certification and requiring recertification every seven years to retain diplomate status. The largest of the specialty boards, the American Board of Internal Medicine, became a pacesetter when it initiated voluntary recertification to retain diplomate status. An impulse to "do the right thing" was seen as a few thousand internists volunteered for recertification. The first exam was given in 1974, but by 1980, only 7600 diplomates had been recertified, less than 10 percent of those who were eligible during this time period. The internal medicine board then adopted a new voluntary approach, the Advanced Achievement in Internal Medicine (AAIM), and used Madison Avenue help to market it, but the first round of achievement exams attracted only 1300 volunteers. And the numbers of volunteers in the other specialties were similarly unimpressive. In fact, no other proposal has raised more anxiety and paranoia than the recertification schemes. The practitioner perceives recertification as a threat to the right to practice and considers it a potential blow to self-esteem. Concerns include expectations of repeating the original certification process, taking another written exam, and worse yet, being held responsible for a large body of knowledge not necessarily related to their practices.

The specialty boards have determined that time-limited certification is the most reasonable approach assuring continued competence. At the end of the period of the certificate, the diplomate must achieve recertification or lose diplomate status. There are some family practitioners who are now on their third cycle, having been certified and twice recertified. Surgery followed and was the first board to interrupt its 40-year practice of issuing permanent certificates when it initiated time-limited certificates in 1976. Today 16 of the 23 boards have established time-limited certification and others are now considering that direction. The American Board of Plastic Surgery, however, reconsidered, and recertification has been eliminated, bringing the total back to 15. Nevertheless, it is safe to predict that most, if not all, boards will, within a few years, require recertification. Although psychiatry is not yet one of the boards to require recertification, such a step will likely be taken at some point. When this occurs, psychiatry will require periodic redefinition in order to do a recertification process every 7 to 10 years. No field in medical science is static, and the very process of recertification recognizes how important it is to deal with those changes.

Changes in the Health Care System

These changes, so widespread that it is difficult to summarize their content or impact in a few words, are discussed at greater length in Chapter 2, by Jonathan F. Borus; here we cite but a few.

Cost reimbursement gives way to competition.   The theme of the new economic approach to health care has been cost containment. For the past half-dozen years, the policy makers have stressed the need to contain the cost of an inflationary health care system. The first major step was the 1983 shift from cost reimbursement for any medically necessary service to a prepaid payment system (PPS), which featured Medicare payments to hospitals on the basis of *diagnosis-related groups* (DRGs). Instead of payment for actual cost, the hospital was reimbursed on a formula basis, with a specific amount for each admission diagnostically categorized into one of the DRG categories. If the case were complicated, if excessive numbers of diagnostic tests or procedures were used, or if the stay were too long, the hospital lost money; if the hospital costs were less than the allowed amount, the hospital could keep the profit. All of this was introduced in an era of competition. To increase their "market-share," institutions and individual practitioners began to cut costs, to advertise, and to try to meet the needs of health care plans. Instead of the solo practitioner style of practice, physicians began to practice in single specialty and multispecialty groups. The initial impetus was to increase the quality of care and to make the life of the physician more convenient. These reasons gave way to focus on economic advantages and attracting business. To attract the attention of those who buy medical services, physicians organized *preferred providers organizations* (PPOs), which offered comprehensive care at discounts. Health care entrepreneurs organized *health maintenance organizations* (HMOs), which featured a combination of preventive services and comprehensiveness of care. Diminished costs were accomplished by tough restrictions on the use of hospital services (the most costly of all health care), and gatekeepers were employed to avoid unnecessary use of subspecialist services. Again, the attraction for third party payers (government, commercial insurance companies, big businesses which established their own health care systems for employees) was reduced cost. The availability of these new systems made competition a motivating force. Even the language changed to that of business and Madison Avenue. Terms like *market share* and *product line* rolled glibly off the tongues of administrators and physicians alike. Initially psychiatry had the advantage of an exclusion from DRGs because of the problems of predicting costs, the diversity of hospital stays for acute and chronic illness in private and public hospitals, and problems in classifying mental disorders.

However, psychiatrists created that exclusion only through careful studies of treatment costs, and there is little doubt that psychiatry will soon fall under the PPS regulations. Psychiatrists have joined other specialists in moving into multispecialty groups and in establishing psychiatric PPOs or joining multi-specialty PPOs. Psychiatrists are adopting a realistic view of the future—a health care delivery system based on competition and ruled by cost containment.

Limited coverage for psychiatric illness. Another change in the health care system is reduced coverage for psychiatric illness. Psychiatry has always been a junior partner in the coverage offered by insurance plans. In part, this is due to tradition—the cost of psychiatric treatment in public-funded institutions has primarily been borne by state and local governments. But it is due also to the stigma associated with mental illness. People are willing to deny their potential need for psychiatric treatment and often prefer to insure themselves against the cost of dental treatment, eyeglass services, or prescription services. The theme of "dental or mental" is proffered by insurers, who are always eager to save the 10 percent of premiums, the ordinary cost of psychiatric care in such plans. The insurer's fear is that the demand for psychiatric treatment will be limitless, a fear reinforced by the increasing numbers of psychotherapy providers (all seeking coverage under insurance plans), and by the unpredictability of costs. Significant limitations on coverage (limited numbers of days in acute care settings, limited numbers of outpatient visits), higher deductibles, and coinsurance payments have been the consequences, along with a shift from long-term psychoanalytically oriented psychotherapy (or formal psychoanalysis) to brief or crisis-oriented psychotherapy and increased use of medication to shorten the duration of illness. Instead of paying for treatment of any psychiatric diagnosis, insurers seek to cover only those conditions causing functional disability and serious symptoms (psychotic disorders) and to disclaim coverage for conditions which are predominantly inhibitions in social interaction or those problems which limit the realization of one's potential. The shift is away from the treatment of personality disorders and symptoms of psychoneuroses except to the extent of dealing with the crises which arise in the lives of those afflicted with such conditions. A profession that in the past spent about 70 percent of its time doing office psychotherapy for personality disorders is shifting its styles of practice to a combination of office and hospital practices, with short-term and crisis-oriented therapies.

Remedicalization

It is popular to describe some of the changes in psychiatric practice as *remedicalization*. Among those who have never abandoned a medical orientation, we prefer to view the change as a shift to a greater emphasis on the *biology* in the *biopsychosocial* orientation of the psychiatrist. Psychiatrists are now more frequently exposed to physicians in other specialties and are more likely to participate in general medical organizations. This is in part a consequence of the shift from separate psychiatric hospitals to treatment in psychiatric units of acute care general hospitals. It is also a result of the increased focus on psychiatric consultation for patients on other medical services whose treatment may be aided by psychiatric expertise or whose reaction to illness may include serious psychiatric symptoms. Another factor influencing this shift includes increased practice in multispecialty groups. Association with other physicians has reinforced the medical identity of the psychiatrist and increased attention to the pathophysiological factors that can produce changes in mental functioning, mood, or behavior. One sad fact remains, however— too many psychiatrists are unwilling to be responsible for the physical examination of patients, partly because of fear that touching the patient will complicate the transference or affect the doctor–patient relationship and partly because of fear that these skills have atrophied. These issues are discussed at greater length by Jeffrey Houpt in Chapter 5.

The Physician Glut

Yager and Borus (1987) have published a challenging review asking whether we are training too many psychiatrists. They suggest that under the present system for training psychiatrists, shifts in demands for services, changing payment and access patterns, increasing numbers of nonpsychiatrist mental health professionals, and a surfeit of primary care physicians will lead to an underemployment of psychiatrists. There is no doubt that an oversupply of physicians is already upon us and that it will be an increasing factor in the health care system, but the effect on psychiatric practice will be to focus more attention on quality. Quality attracts attention when there is a buyer's market, and it often slips when suppliers are short. Hopefully, the Residency Review Committee in psychiatry will more rigorously enforce general and special requirements and thus improve quality. As noted earlier in this chapter, recertification will probably be instituted in the form of time-limited certification, and new performance-assessment techniques will allow recertification to be based on performance, rather than simply repeating a cognitive examination. Reregistration of licensure will also require competency assessment, and New York State has already circulated a proposal calling for such assessment as a condition of relicensure. Performance assessed according to national standards motivates psychiatrists to update their knowledge and to alter their styles of practice to factor in new treatments.

The Definition of a Psychiatrist

Formerly, a psychiatrist was pronounced competent by the successful completion of an accredited residency program. The special requirements for residency accreditation define what must and should be taught in accredited programs. From that criterion, a psychiatrist becomes one whose definition depends on training.

Another definition for a psychiatrist is one who has become certified as a specialist in psychiatry by the American Board of Psychiatry and Neurology (ABPN) by passing a two-part examination. Part I of the examination tests basic knowledge; part II, an oral exam, focuses on skills, judgment, and attitudes. Even more desirable would be to define a psychiatrist in terms of the measurable skills and knowledge deemed necessary by teachers and practitioners in the field. A number of attempts to define educational objectives have been published. They range from those developed by Yager and Pasnau (1976) at the University of California in Los Angeles, to a comprehensive and detailed list published by Thompson (1979). Using the *critical incident* technique, in which data were collected from practitioners, the Committee on Certification in Child Psychiatry (1976) of the ABPN developed a list of realistic practice skills for child psychiatrists.

An Operational Approach

One useful approach to definition is to take an operational view of a psychiatrist, a task analysis if you will! This assumes that what psychiatrists do creates the current definition of the field. If a psychiatrist is to be defined in operational terms, and if the field is to be so described, it is essential to decide what body of knowledge must be mastered, what skills acquired, and what attitudes expressed (Langsley and Hollender, 1982). But will that definition remain constant?

Langsley and Hollender (1982) conducted a survey of teachers and practitioners to obtain a description of the educational ideals and practice patterns, current in 1980, that define a psychiatrist. A questionnaire asking them to rate the skills, knowledge, and attitudes a specialist in psychiatry should possess was circulated to 430 full-time academicians and 430 practitioners (a random sample of APA members who were not salaried academicians). There was a 70 percent response rate from the teachers and a 43 percent rate from the practitioners, yielding a total of 482 responses. Data analysis consisted of identifying the skills and knowledge chosen most frequently by a large proportion of the respondents. More than 50 percent of respondents voted to include 23 of the 32 skill items, and 24 of the knowledge items were so rated by 75 percent of respondents. The attitudinal descriptors did not distinguish the psychiatrist from other physicians because they were too general. They included such dimensions as ethical conduct, commitment to maintaining competency, responsibility to patients, and other virtues.

From the knowledge and skill items commonly regarded as important, Langsley and Hollender constructed a model of the psychiatrist of that vintage. The skills were categorized under evaluation, treatment, personality of the psychiatrist, and record-keeping and forensic skills. The descriptions ranked highest fell in the evaluation group and included skills such as interviewing, evaluating the need for hospitalization, making diagnoses, assessing suicidal or homicidal potential, fomulating the problems of patients referred for consultation, using laboratory tests, and other skills related to the comprehensive evaluation of the patient. Treatment skills were also very highly ranked, the most important being developing a treatment plan and implementing it. Other key treatment skills included the ability to do supportive psychotherapy and the use of psychoactive drugs. Highly ranked items describing the personality of the psychiatrist included reliability, integrity, interest in patients, recognition of countertransference problems, and objectivity.

In the list of knowledge items, evaluation and treatment were again regarded as the most important descriptors of a psychiatrist. Evaluation was the category for such high-ranking items as knowledge of treatment, use of medication and certain types of psychotherapy. Insight therapy was considered far less important than supportive psychotherapy.

Both teachers and practitioners defined a *specialist in psychiatry* as a clinician whose principal skills were in evaluating and treating psychiatric disorder. The psychiatrist functions as a generalist concerned with medication, hospitalization, supportive psychotherapy, and occasionally family or group therapy or ECT. The psychiatrist was differentiated from other mental health professionals who do only psychotherapy. One could ask how the psychiatrist who does only psychotherapy differs from nonpsychiatric psychotherapists, but, to be defined as a specialist in psychiatry, the physician had to possess other skills and knowledge of a psychiatrist, whether they were used often or not. The psychiatrist was expected to know a great deal about differential diagnosis of various syndromes, the management of psychiatric emergencies, the ability to treat patients in a hospital, psychodynamic formulations, and consultation. Basic skills involved the practice and theory of the use of medications and psychotherapies. Children were not seen as a responsibility of the general psychiatrist, and individual patients were regarded as more important than a family or group. Direct work with patients ranked much higher than community psychiatry or administration.

Langsley and Yager (1988) replicated the 1980 study. The replication was done because the changes in psychiatric practice were assumed to have altered general agreement on the skills and knowledge defining a specialist in psychiatry. A questionnaire was circulated to the 355 members of the American Association of Directors of Psychiatric Residency Training and to the 130 members of the American Association of Chairmen of Departments of Psychiatry, as well as to 499 full-time practitioners. There were 257 responses from teachers and 223 from practitioners. The 480 responses in 1987 were compared with the 482 responses from the 1980 survey. With the exception of 10 new knowledge items and 16 new skill items, the questions were the same in both as in the 1980 projects (see Tables 1, 2, 3, and 4). In addition, respondents were asked to rate whether each topic should be considered an important aspect of a psychiatric subspecialty.

Fifteen of the skill items had an agreement rating of more than 90 percent, and 20 of the knowledge items had a similar high level (greater than 90 percent) of agreement. There were both similarities and differences between the 1980 and 1987 results: As in 1980, the high-agreement list of skills fell

Table 1. Skills That Psychiatrists Should Possess as Agreed Upon by 85 Percent or More of Respondents to the 1980 Survey

Psychiatrists should be able to:

- Conduct comprehensive psychiatric interviews
- Conduct diagnostic family interviews
- Consistently demonstrate interest, tact, and compassion for patients and their families
- Demonstrate reliability, conscientiousness, and integrity
- Remain objective, keeping a professional stance, be neither too distant nor too involved
- Use appropriate laboratory tests, psychological tests, and other diagnostic procedures
- Make accurate psychiatric diagnoses
- Formulate problem lists and corresponding treatment plans and implement them personally or through appropriate referrals
- Evaluate the need for hospitalization
- Conduct crisis intervention
- Conduct brief psychotherapy
- Provide supportive psychotherapy, with awareness of psychodynamic issues
- Recognize countertransference problems and personal idiosyncrasies, when they influence interactions with patients, and deal with them constructively
- Use psychopharmacological agents effectively
- Maintain adequate records, including history, mental status, physical examination, diagnostic tests, and notes indicating the progress of treatment
- Develop liaison relationships with physicians, nurses, and social workers
- Construct comprehensive assessments of the problems of physically ill or psychosomatically ill patients referred for consultation and communicate the results to the referring physician, with practical suggestions for management
- Undertake the psychiatric treatment of patients with psychophysiological or physical illnesses
- Work harmoniously in mental health teams to gather information, plan treatments, and implement treatments
- Assess and treat/manage psychiatric problems of the aged
- Assess and treat/manage alcoholism
- Assess and treat/manage sedative/psychostimulant abuse
- Assess and treat/manage eating disorders
- Assess developmental and psychopathological problems of adolescents (Note: Only 74 percent of respondents agreed that all psychiatrists should be able to conduct psychotherapy with adolescents)

under the categories of evaluation, treatment, personality of the psychiatrist, and record keeping. An *assess, treat/manage* category for certain conditions had been added, and many achieved high rankings. Of the 25 most highly ranked items, eight fell under the category of evaluation, six under treatment, five under personality of the psychiatrist, four under assess, treat/manage certain conditions, and one under record keeping. Evaluation and treatment skills

Table 2. Other Skills Important for the General Psychiatrist from the 1987 Survey

I. Skills believed to be required by 70 percent to 85 percent of respondents:
   1. Assess suicidal and homicidal potential or potential for assaultive behavior
   2. Perform a competent physical examination including a detailed neurological examination
   3. Conduct a neurobehavioral assessment
   4. Assess and treat/manage narcotics abuse
   5. Assess and treat/manage sexual dysfunction
   6. Teach knowledge and skills appropriate to psychiatry to colleagues and medical students
   7. Conduct outpatient family or marital therapy
   8. Conduct inpatient and/or outpatient group psychotherapy
   9. Conduct psychotherapy with adolescents
   10. Demonstrate proficiency in psychoanalytically oriented psychotherapy
   11. Conduct cognitive therapy
   12. Conduct psychotherapeutic treatment of dying patients
   13. Administer psychiatric treatment programs

II. Skills believed necessary for psychiatrists by 50 percent to 70 percent of respondents:
   1. Conduct thorough evaluation of children and their families when a child is the identified patient
   2. Conduct forensic evaluations and give testimony on issues such as mental competency, sanity, and compensation for psychological and mental injury
   3. Comprehensively manage psychiatric problems of patients with epilepsy, brain injury, and other structural brain abnormalities
   4. Administer ECT
   5. Conduct behavior modification therapy
   6. Assess and treat/manage mental retardation
   7. Conduct interventions appropriate to preventive psychiatry at the community level

III. Skills believed necessary by less than 50 percent of respondents:
   1. Conduct play therapy
   2. Conduct psychiatric research
   3. Conduct hypnotic interviews for diagnostic purposes

were ranked highest. Items describing the personality of the psychiatrist achieved higher rankings than in the 1980 study. Five of the top 25 included items describing the ability to recognize countertransference problems and personal idiosyncrasies; the ability to demonstrate interest, tact and compassion; the ability to remain objective; the ability to be reliable; and the ability to work harmoniously as a member of a team. Most of these items were evaluated in importance in 1987. Certain evaluation skills dropped in ranking, especially the items calling for the ability to formulate a problem list and treatment plan. The ability to evaluate children dropped from rank order

Table 3. Knowledge That Psychiatrists Should Possess as Agreed Upon by 85 Percent or More of Respondents to the 1987 Survey

Psychiatrists should be able to knowledgeably discuss the following:

- Principles of ethics related to psychiatry
- Merits and limitations of scientific literature
- Criteria for differentiating organic and functional disorders
- Nosology and classification of mental disorders, including childhood disorders
- Differential diagnosis of psychiatric syndromes
- Descriptive psychiatry, including various clinical syndromes
- Basic concepts of psychiatric epidemiology
- Characteristics of and explanations for psychotic, neurotic, characterologic, and borderline disorders
- Psychological aspects of stress, coping, and adaptation, including dying, bereavement, and other life crises
- Specific syndromes in consultation psychiatry
- Indications for and limitations of psychological assessment
- Principles of human growth and development, including major theories and biopsychosocial considerations
- Basic psychoanalytic concepts and theories
- Common psychiatric problems of childhood
- Adolescence, with focus on personality developmental theories
- Basic concepts of group dynamics
- Basic concepts of family organization and communication
- Principles for evaluating children and their families
- Genetic and dynamic formulations, including precipitating stresses, interpersonal relationships, character structure, psychodynamics, and effects of illness on others
- Neurobiological basic sciences
- Physiology of sleep and sleep disturbances
- Major biochemical theories of psychopathology
- Major theories of addiction
- Psychiatrically pertinent aspects of neurology
- Forensic psychiatry, including patients' rights, commitment, privileged communication, testamentary capacity, and competency
- Evaluation and management of psychiatric emergencies
- Indications and contraindications for hospitalization
- Theories of therapy, indications and contraindications, basic assumptions, and data about outcome
- Principles of intervention in child and adolescent psychiatry
- Indications and contraindications for various types of psychotherapy (individual, family, marital, social)
- Psychoanalytically oriented psychotherapy
- Family therapy
- Group therapy
- Indications, contraindications, presumed mechanisms, dosing schedules, and side effects for common psychopharmacological agents
- Indications, contraindications, and theories regarding mechanism of action of ECT
- Principles of evaluation and intervention in geriatric psychiatry
- Psychosomatic theories on pathogenesis and evaluation and therapies of psychosomatic disorders
- Models of consultation and liaison psychiatry

Table 4. Other Knowledge Important for the General Psychiatrist from the 1987 Survey

1. Seventy to 85 percent of respondents agreed that the general psychiatrist should be able to knowledgeably discuss the following:

- Basic principles of learning theories
- Basic concepts of social psychiatry
- Principles of preventive psychiatry at the community and clinical levels
- Psychiatric problems of specific ethnic and underprivileged populations
- Mental retardation including evaluation and treatment planning
- Community mental health including consultation and program evaluation
- History of psychiatry
- Psychotherapies: couples therapy, cognitive therapies, behavior modification

2. Sixty-two to 70 percent of respondents agreed that the general psychiatrist should be able to knowledgeably discuss the following:

- Psychotherapies: child psychotherapy
- Psychiatric economics: patterns of private and public funding, reimbursement
- Principles of psychiatric administration

number 23 to number 39, and forensic evaluation dropped from rank number 24 to number 40.

Certain treatment skills were either more highly ranked or, when added to the list of new items, achieved very high rankings. Examples are the ability to do crisis intervention and the ability to do brief psychotherapy. Supportive psychotherapy continued to be the highest of the treatment skills and the ability to use psychopharmacological agents dropped slightly, from rank number 8 to number 12. Proficiency in psychoanalytically oriented psychotherapy was very low (number 36) in 1987, as it had been in 1980. By contrast, supportive therapy, crisis intervention, and brief psychotherapy were ranked very highly.

Knowledge required of a specialist in psychiatry paralleled the required skills. The top 20 knowledge items included nine related to evaluation, three to treatment, one to the personality of the psychiatrist, four to specific syndromes, and three to an area that might be called *basic psychology*. The items ranked as more important in 1987 include indications for psychological assessment, knowledge about common psychiatric problems of children, and knowledge of the evaluation of children. Note, however, that, although knowledge about children was highly ranked, the ability to treat children was not regarded as essential to the general psychiatrist.

Those knowledge items considered less important in 1987 were genetic and dynamic formulations (which dropped from rank number 8 to number 16), growth and development (which dropped from number 9 to number 18), psychoanalytically oriented psychotherapy (which dropped from number 12 to number 27) and group therapy, family therapy, couples therapy, behavior modification, and child therapy.

Subspecialization in Psychiatry

Subspecialization, which will be discussed in detail in Chapter 4, has become a reality in psychiatry (Yager and Langsley, 1987). Though only one area is recognized by a formal credential (child psychiatry), increasing numbers of psychiatrists have taken postresidency fellowships in subspecialty areas and focus their practices on a limited field. The debate about subspecialization and the need for credentialing subspecialists prompted Langsley and Yager to include questions about subspecialization in the 1987 replication. Respondents were asked whether each skill and knowledge item should be considered part of a subspecialty. More than 50 percent of the respondents felt that a total of nine skill items and 11 knowledge items were important aspects of some psychiatric subspecialties. The content of those items suggested that the subspecialties include child psychiatry, adolescent psychiatry, psychoanalysis, geropsychiatry, forensic psychiatry, consultation/liaison psychiatry, alcohol and drug dependence psychiatry, and administrative psychiatry. These definitions were not considered a sensitive measure of the specific content in each field, only a gross estimate of the importance of subspecialties. Further studies of the required knowledge and skills in the subspecialties should be accomplished with respondents skilled in the specific subspecialties under study. The ABPN has now applied for authorization to issue subspecialty certificates in geriatric psychiatry.

These are inevitable trends and not only is increased subspecialization likely, but it will probably carry with it the possibility of upgrading the quality of psychiatric practice and education. In fact, subspecialization may render psychiatry even more competitive in relation to other mental health care providers. It is not necessary to assume that subspecialization will render general psychiatry obsolete; psychiatric subspecialties superimposed on the fundamental skills of general psychiatry should enable practitioners to better help a greater variety of patients and associated professions.

What Is a Psychiatrist?

The definition of *psychiatrist* will change as psychiatric science advances and new methods of psychiatric practice are influenced by economic issues. The psychiatrist of tomorrow is more likely to be a subspecialist, as well as a generalist, and is likely to be required to be recertified periodically. The psychiatrist of today is more likely to be involved with patients with the more severe disorders, and they are likely to focus on techniques that are more classically medical. The psychotherapy practiced by tomorrow's psychiatrist is more likely to be brief and crisis-oriented, not long-term and insight-oriented. Only one prediction is safe—tomorrow's psychiatrist will be different than today's.

References

Langsley DG, Hollender MH: The definition of a psychiatrist. Am J Psychiatry 1982; 139:81–85

Langsley DG, Yager J: The definition of a psychiatrist: a decade later. Am J Psychiatry 1988; 145:469–475

McDermott JF, McGuire C, Berner ES: Roles and functions of child psychiatrists. Evanston, IL, American Board of Psychiatry and Neurology, 1976

Thompson MGG: A Resident's Guide to Psychiatric Education. New York, Plenum Press, 1979

Yager J, Borus JF: Are we training too many psychiatrists? Am J Psychiatry 1987; 144:1042–1048

Yager J, Langsley DG: The evolving subspecialization of psychiatry: implications for the profession. Am J Psychiatry 1987; 1461–1465

Yager J, Pasnau RO: The educational objectives of a psychiatric residency program. Am J Psychiatry 1976; 133:217–220

Chapter 2

How Will New Practice Settings Change Psychiatry?

Jonathan F. Borus, M.D.

Dramatic changes are forecast for medical care systems and physician practice settings in the near future. We have witnessed the rapid growth of managed health care in health maintenance organizations, preferred provider organizations, and for-profit health chains, and we have seen the impact of these settings on the practice activities of their physicians. In the coming decade, all signs point to a radical shift in the organization of health care that is likely to both influence psychiatrists' lives and direct their professional activities.

The Economy and Health Care

One underlying reason for such changes is the enormous cost to the nation of health care. Health costs, temporarily plateaued by diagnosis-related groups (DRGs), are again rising at an alarming rate at a time when the country is facing huge budget deficits (Costs of health care, 3 April 1987, p. 17). Economists and politicians tell us we will have to find methods that ration health care, to cap its cost. Lester Thurow, a Massachusetts Institute of Technology Sloan School health economist, attributes the current dilemma to a nation in conflict between capitalist and egalitarian values that make it hard to ration care (Thurow, 1984). Capitalistic values spur technological innovations in medicine, with the development of exciting but very expensive ways to treat patients that often focus on prolonging the final portions of life; egalitarian values encourage us to demand that these expensive innovations be made available to all, regardless of their ability to pay for them. Thurow (1984) points out that we will soon reach a point where we cannot afford to go the "extra mile" for every patient regardless of cost. The onus is on the medical profession to prove that the marginal benefits accrued to the patient exceed the additional costs of providing the new treatments and that what we do, at extra cost, makes a meaningful difference (Thurow, 1985). In the absence of such proof, Thurow believes economic factors will dominate; this will lead to rationing based on uncoordinated development of a three-tiered health care system that provides differential access to care. The lowest tier will be funded by the government at a *safety-net level*, in which the indigent will receive health care from a designated provider-organization that is compensated on a per capita basis for all illnesses occurring within a specific period of time. The second tier is also likely to be a capitated system, subsidized by industry, that will provide a level of care, as an employment benefit, higher than the government safety net. The third tier will be additional care, above capitated benefits, available to individuals willing to pay for it out-of-pocket; obviously, this higher level of care will be available only to those with independent means.

Organized/Managed Health Care Systems

To provide such capitated care, the forecasters predict that a small number (perhaps 10 to 20 in total) of *supermed systems*—owned and operated by insurers, for-profit chains, and perhaps teaching hospitals—will control most of the health care in this country by 1995 (American Psychiatric Association, 1986). The hospital itself will become too expensive a setting to provide the care it does now, and there will be increasing pressure to use less expensive care alternatives (American College of Hospital Administrators, 1984; Health Insurance Association of America, 1985). The supermed care systems will diversify to include not only hospitals, but also a variety of outpatient treatment centers, rehabilitation centers, nursing homes, day treatment facilities, and their own primary care practices, including health maintenance organizations (HMOs), preferred provider organizations (PPOs), EPOs, IPAs, and other group practices. These supermed systems will be developed for both clinical and economic reasons, and, by linking facilities for all aspects of a patient's care needs closely into one network, they will best be able to meet the fiscal requirement of providing the least expensive alternative meeting the patient's needs, thereby keeping the system's costs competitive.

One corollary of these events is the likelihood that the solo private practice of medicine will decrease dramatically or perhaps become extinct (Abramowitz, 1985). Solo practices will be too expensive and unable to provide competitive capitated care. Most physicians are therefore likely to work as members of managed health care systems, either as salaried employees or as subcontractors providing care at discounted or decreased fees. In either situation, physicians will find their autonomy lessened by their dependence on the health care system (Gurevitz, 1984). These forecasters also predict an oversupply of physicians and other health care providers, all trying to seize the largest piece of the most profitable third-tier care for those who can pay for extra services (Issue of physician supply, 24 Jan 1986, p. 31). In such a situation, individual physicians and health care systems not able to provide cost-effective, financially competitive care may well go out of business (Ginzberg, 1985; Petersdorf, 1985).

Impact on Psychiatrists

Fewer Psychiatrists Will Be Needed

What impact will changes in the organization and settings of medical care have on psychiatrists and psychiatric care? First, it is highly likely that there will be an excess of psychiatrists relative to what the new medical marketplace can afford or utilize (Yager and Borus, 1987). Indeed, some urban areas are already saturated with psychiatrists, and the current ratio of 15 psychiatrists per 100,000 population is well within health-planner estimates of provider need. Our current graduating rate, from 1000 to 1200 new psychiatrists each year, should easily meet the Graduate Medical Education National Advisory Council (GMENAC) projection of psychiatric need by 1990. However, the GMENAC projections were overly generous because they did not take into consideration the multiple economic and care system changes discussed above.

In addition, psychiatrists face increasing competition in the mental health market from psychologists, social workers, nurses, and the rapid proliferation of masters-level generic therapists. These groups are growing at faster rates, clustering in the same geographic areas, and willingly taking on less desirable jobs and sicker patients, at lower rates of pay than psychiatrists. Within an increasingly cost-conscious health market, we are being undersold and the demand for psychiatric services, especially psychotherapy, has already been sharply affected by these less expensive, albeit perhaps lower quality, therapists. Capitated, managed-care systems, striving to provide care as inexpensively as possible and make a profit, are likely to preferentially employ these less costly mental health providers, as has happened in HMOs and mental health centers, and the demand and need for psychiatrists is likely to decrease (Feldman and Goldman, 1986). To survive in such systems, psychiatrists must learn to market what they do better than others; one viewer of the changing medical and mental health scene has suggested that the concept of *market or morbidity* will become the analog of the *publish or perish* imperative in academia (Cummings and Duhl, 1986).

The Psychiatrist's Role and Functions Will Change

As per capita mechanisms are put into place, integrated systems of psychiatric care will be needed to link traditional hospitalization and outpatient therapy with general medical care, partial hospitalization, nursing-home care, sheltered-living facilities, residential treatment centers, and other services if economical and competitive care is to be provided for individuals throughout the course of illness. As most psychiatrists will probably work in these integrated systems, the organization and needs of the new systems will affect what the psychiatrists of the future will do. To prove that psychiatry offers unique services unavailable from other professionals, psychiatry will move toward greater subspecialization; subspecialization will also be used to justify psychiatrists' higher charges. The psychiatrist will less frequently be the primary psychotherapist, as less expensive mental health professionals can do that work, and will more usually be medical, psychoanalytic, or behaviorally oriented consultants to nonpsychiatric primary therapists and general physicians. Although subspecialists, we hopefully will remain the expert diagnosticians in these settings because of our comprehensive knowledge of the potential medical, neurological, and psychological components of a patient's illness.

Psychiatrists in such settings must also be more familiar with short-term, behaviorally oriented interventions, not aiming to foster structural or characterologic change. In a competitive market if such brief, inexpensive interventions can alleviate current symptoms, most consumers and care systems will select them as the psychiatric benefit package of choice. In longitudinal work at the Kaiser Health Plan, Cummings and Duhl (1986) report that 85 percent of patients were most interested in, satisfied with, and felt helped by short-term therapy; they suggest that future cost-conscious patients, when bargaining for mental health and other benefits, will be willing to pay only for the short-term therapies. Psychotherapy by psychiatrists may return to the third-tier carriage trade, paid for out-of-pocket as it was prior to insurance coverage for outpatient psychotherapy. But it is unlikely that this third tier will be able to support anywhere near the 56 percent of psychiatrists in private practice in the mid-1980s (Fenton, 1987). Great competition with the multitude of other, less expensive psychotherapists for this most profitable out-of-pocket care can also be expected.

Constraints on Psychiatrists in Health Care Systems

In addition to changing what we do, there may be major changes in how we do it. Psychiatrists employed by managed care systems will have decreased autonomy in determining what they do and when and how long they do it in caring for their patients. The providers, as well as their care, will be *managed*, with great pressure to increase *productivity* and with the potential for care quality to suffer under the stress of providing a higher quantity of care. Increased productivity demands are likely to decrease time for research and academic work, and this could lead to professional isolation. There may also be changes in the psychiatrist's incentives and allegiances. A salaried physician has less incentive to provide continuing care to a difficult patient or to put the patient's needs above those of the care system. With its competitive nature, the system's emphasis will be on "keeping the customers happy," something that psychiatrists are not always able to do when, as part of therapy, they withhold gratification. Treatment will be dictated by resource availability and care may be either discouraged or denied if defined benefits end. The result will be more patients forced into the first-tier, public-sector system (Schiff et al., 1986).

These managed care systems will operate under a gatekeeper concept, in which primary physicians channel and sanction all specialist care (Feldman and Goldman, 1986). The gatekeepers, operating under fiscal incentives to limit the amount of specialist care, will therefore determine whom the psychiatrist sees and at what stage of illness. This gatekeeping system is also likely to insure that most patient triage will be performed by generalists who, many studies have shown, are not proficient at recognizing and diagnosing mental disorder (Hoeper, 1979). Psychiatrists will be used as consultants to the gatekeepers, and they will often be asked to cover the gatekeeper's work and that of other primary therapists. As community mental health center psychiatrists have found, other managed-care psychiatrists will need to develop care standards and to specify what they will cover and what they won't, as in not signing prescriptions unless the psychiatrist has directly evaluated the patient (G. Clark, unpublished data, 1988). Even with such standards, psychiatrists will often find themselves harnessed by substantial medicolegal responsibilities, paired with management constraints on their authority. Since many of these issues have already arisen in today's for-profit hospitals, HMOs, and community mental health centers, the APA set up a Task Force on Psychiatric Practice Issues in Organized/Managed Care Settings, which is exploring the psychiatrist's role in such settings and making suggestions to improve it.

Implications for Psychiatric Training and Research

These many projected changes in the practice of psychiatry should alert us to a need to make changes in today's training of tomorrow's psychiatrists. It appears obvious there should be greater stress on learning short-term behavioral and cognitive therapies and psychopharmacologic interventions, which relieve symptoms on a time-limited, cost-effective basis. We will have to train our residents to be better consultants to, and supervisors of, less expensive mental health professionals and primary care general physician gatekeepers; the latter training should occur not only in tertiary hospital settings, but also through rotations in primary care settings. Training should put a higher premium on the retention of medical and neurologic knowledge, as well as the development of psychologic skills, so that the psychiatrist has the breadth of knowledge needed to maintain the role of expert diagnostician. Finally, we will need to provide some advanced training in actual managed-care settings, to allow residents to learn how to practice most effectively in them.

A potential benefit of these changes is that competitive managed-care settings must emphasize effectiveness. The onus will be on us in the future to show that we provide essential care that others can't and that our care makes a difference in the life and health of the patient. Investigations such as the Rand Corporation's National Study of Medical Outcomes, which is comparing utilization, cost, clinical outcomes, and satisfaction for patients with major depression treated in variously structured organizational health care settings by providers of different disciplines, will give us one type of useful information about who does what best, where, and how. In addition, randomized off-set studies, which compare the cost, utilization, and clinical outcomes of patients with similar mental disorders randomly assigned for treatment to mental health specialists and general health providers (who in future gate-keeper systems are expected to provide an even higher percentage of the nation's mental health care), will help us define those disorders and situations for which our extra cost is warranted by superior results. The sooner we embark on such studies, the stronger will be our bargaining and marketing position when we press for the inclusion and high valuation of psychiatrists in managed-care systems. As the findings of such studies can strongly influence what psychiatrists are allowed to do in the practice settings of the future, in this area, as in few others, our fate is in our own hands.

References

Abramowitz KS: The future of health care delivery in America. New York, NY, Bernstein Research, Sanford C. Bernstein & Co., 1985

American College of Hospital Administrators: Health care in the 1990s: trends and strategies. Chicago, IL, Arthur Anderson & Co., 1984

American Psychiatric Association Office of Economic Affairs: Status report on developments in the health care industry. Washington, DC, American Psychiatric Association, 1986

Costs of health care rose seven times faster in 1986 than costs of other goods, services. Psychiatric News, 3 April 1987, p 17

Cummings N, Duhl LJ: The new delivery system. Psychiatric Annals 1986; 16:470–475

Feldman S, Goldman B: Mental health care in HMOs: practice and potential. Psychiatric Annals 1986; 16:463–469

Fenton W: Professional activities of psychiatrists, in The Nation's Psychiatrists: 1983 Survey. Washington, DC, American Psychiatric Press, Inc., 1987

Ginzberg E: What lies ahead for American physicians: one economist's view. JAMA 1985; 253:2878–2879

Gurevitz H: Psychiatry and preferred provider organizations. Psychiatric Annals 1984; 14:342–349

Health Insurance Association of America: The health care system in the mid-1990's. Arthur D. Little, Inc., 1985

Hoeper EW: Observations on the impact of psychiatric disorder upon primary medical care, in Institute of Medicine Series on Mental Health Services in General Health Care, volume I. Washington, DC, National Academy of Sciences, 1979

Issue of physician supply merits close attention. American Medical News, 24 January 1986, p 31

Petersdorf RG: Current and future directions for hospital and physician reimbursement. JAMA 1985; 253:2543–2548

Schiff RL, Ansell DA, Schlosser JE, et al: Transfers to a public hospital. N Engl J Med 1986; 314:552–557

Thurow LC: Learning to say "no." N Engl J Med 1984; 311:1569–1572

Thurow LC: Medicine versus economics. N Engl J Med 1985; 313:611–614

Yager J, Borus JF: Are we training too many psychiatrists? Am J Psychiatry 1987; 144:1042–1048

Chapter 3

The Future Psychiatrist as a Generalist: Arguments Against Credentials for Subspecialists

Sidney H. Weissman, M.D.
Philip G. Bashook, Ed.D.

The development of medicine in the United States during this century has seen major shifts in the nature of medical training, medical practice, and medical research. The Flexner report (1910) is credited with moving medical education from an investor-owned education model to its current position in the mainstream of academia. By 1920, medical schools as part of major universities had become well established, with full-time faculty and thriving research laboratories (Ludmerer, 1985). Changes in the stature of the medical school did not, in and of themselves, alter the practice of medicine; however, the scientific revolution and the knowledge explosion since the turn of the century are some of the most important forces for the dramatic change in medicine and the proliferation of specialties.

Starting with the general practitioner, who provided basic medical care at the turn of the century, we now have a vast array of physicians and surgeons with specialized knowledge and technical expertise to provide care. Assuring the public of the professional expertise of physicians and setting standards of practice has been orchestrated by two separate but related credentialing procedures. A legal credential, in the form of the basic license to practice medicine in the United States, is controlled by individual states. The second credentialing process is certification in specialties. Organizations of physicians have assumed responsibility for designating medical specialties and credentialing individuals as specialists. This chapter will concentrate on the latter credentialing process and particularly the issue of credentialing subspecialists.

Today we accept the existence of medical specialists and the credentialing mechanism of certifying boards to formally recognize medical specialists and subspecialists. Historically, the question at issue has not been whether there should be specialists, but rather how to proceed with credentialing them. Recognition through credentialing began in 1917, with certificates of specialization in ophthalmology. Yet the umbrella organization of specialty boards, the American Board of Medical Specialties (ABMS), was founded only 54 years ago. Prominent certifying boards were started in the 1930's. The American Board of Psychiatry and Neurology was founded in 1935, and the American Board of Internal Medicine was started one year later. Thus, recognition of medical specialists is a recent addition to American medicine.

Credentialing of subspecialists is an even more recent event. There are two classifications of board certification designating subspecialization: Certificates of *special qualifications* and certificates of *added qualifications*. Special qualifications are awarded to physicians who successfully complete the general certification requirement, a two-year or longer fellowship program, and an examination in the area of subspecialization. The earliest certificates for subspecialization (special qualifications) were awarded in 1941 by the American Board of Internal Medicine to internists who specialized in pulmonary medicine, gastroenterology, or cardiology. Of the 41 certificates of special qualifications approved by the ABMS and awarded by specialty boards, 29 have been introduced since 1972. The only certificate of special qualification in psychiatry is for child psychiatry, first offered in 1959. Also, not all medical specialty boards have established certificates of special qualifications. Among the 24 member boards of ABMS, six have refrained from credentialing subspecialists.

In 1985, the designation *added qualifications* was created by the ABMS. Although certain procedural questions still need to be worked out, this designation of subspecialization is intermediate between general and special qualifications. Physicians who, after receiving certification as a specialist, undertake prescribed training in a postresidency fellowship program for one or two years, become eligible to sit for a subspecialty examination. Upon successful completion of the exam, the subspecialist will receive a certificate of added qualifications. Currently, there are certificates of special qualifications or added qualifications designated by combined ABMS member boards for hand surgery (American Boards of Anesthesiology, Internal Medicine, Psychiatry and Neurology, Plastic Surgery, General Surgery, and Orthopedic Surgery), critical care medicine (American Boards of Neurological Surgery, Obstetrics and Gynecology, and General Surgery), and geriatric medicine (American Boards of Family Practice and Internal Medicine).

Recently, the American Board of Psychiatry and Neurology has been asked to consider creating a certificate of added qualification in geriatric psychiatry. To consider this request, the American Board of Psychiatry and Neurology has created a task force of board members, psychiatrists, and other physicians to assess the desirability of creating a certificate of added qualification in geriatric psychiatry. If the Board votes to develop added qualifications in a geriatric psychiatry subspecialty, the proposal will be sent to the ABMS for their review and approval. Assuming no major obstacles arise to the development of an added qualification certificate, the final approval of the new certificate would occur in late 1989 or 1990.

The arguments in support of subspecialization are identical to the original argument for specialization: Subspecialization would assert to the public that having good medical care requires physicians with specialized and focused experience, and such expertise is possible only by limiting the focus of clinical expertise. In addition to assuring competency for the public, subspecialization provides clear economic benefits for the practitioner. In today's economic environment, subspecialists are able to charge and receive higher fees for their services. Also, for the academic physicians, subspecialization has an important benefit—the added credentials of subspecialization help define the scope of expertise required to select experts to serve in peer review panels for competitive research grants.

In juxtaposition to the historical trend and the above arguments for credentialing subspecialists in psychiatry, we propose that, at this time, American psychiatry will be better served by not credentialing additional subspecialties in psychiatry.

Clearly, a significant number of subspecialties in psychiatry in addition to child psychiatry have emerged in the past 10 years. Psychiatric subspecialties recognized through formal fellowship programs and/or certification procedures include eating disorders, alcohol and substance abuse, affective disorders, psychopharmacology, forensic psychiatry, administrative psychiatry, psychiatric research, adolescent psychiatry, and geriatric psychiatry. Special knowledge and skills are obviously essential to practice effectively in each of these disciplines. But the important question is, does the development of formal credentialing processes for subspecialties enhance or inhibit the maturation of these disciplines and the quality of psychiatry as a specialty? We contend that, because of the unique nature of organized psychiatry and the multidimensional character of psychiatric practice, altering the current credentialing process for subspecialists will inhibit the natural evolution of subspecialties; it will not stimulate the growth of psychiatry.

Our proposal will be organized around four points:

1. The boundaries of medical specialties and subspecialties are shifting and they will continue to shift.
2. The boundaries and basic core knowledge and skills of a psychiatrist are in dispute.
3. We challenge the argument that psychiatry should follow the model of subspecialty certification utilized in internal medicine
4. We propose using a conceptual framework, based on general systems theory, that provides a way to integrate the sciences of psychology, neuroscience, and social psychology as a foundation for psychiatry.

Guidelines for Subspecialization

A number of guidelines have evolved for the establishment of medical specialties (American Board of Medical Specialties, 1987; Yager et al., 1987). First, a given specialty must have a clear body of knowledge or require special skills. Second, to learn the body of knowledge or attain the skills requires an extensive period of clinical training under careful supervision. Third, there are individuals (specialists) who represent a unique expertise in the medical community and to the lay public, and who are superior in their treatment or diagnostic competence, compared to nonspecialists. Fourth, practitioners in a given specialty tend to define their expertise by discrete paradigm and epistemological borders. The borders of the discipline are codified in specialty journals and books, and through themes at scientific meetings. Scientists define their research agendas and form societies built upon common paradigms of the specialty. Although advances or changes occur, most specialists discourage nonspecialists from practicing in their area of expertise.

Boundary Between Specialty and Subspecialty

In recent years many advances in the basic sciences have been translated into new medical technologies that blur distinctions between medical specialties. Two significant technological developments come to mind. First, in the treatment of cardiac disease, advances in surgical techniques over the past 10 years have established coronary artery bypass surgery as a major surgical procedure and preferred treatment for coronary artery disease. This advance has propelled the growth of cardiovascular (thoracic) surgery as a distinct subspecialty.

In counterpoint to the growth of thoracic surgery, the development of angioplasty has offered the cardiologist a surgical option for treating coronary artery disease. Using angioscopic technology, a cardiologist can treat certain lesions of cardiac vessels without referring the patient to a surgeon (Salem et al., 1987). Both advances in medical technology have led to competition between two distinct subspecialties, cardiology and thoracic surgery, for surgical treatment of the same disease (Dorros and Janke, 1985; Reeder et al., 1986). Both subspecialties claim unique expertise and historical priority. To further complicate this competition, radiologists may, in the future, argue that they and not the cardiologist are best prepared to perform angioplasty because imaging techniques are essential to angioplasty and within the provence of radiology. Clearly, technological advances have changed the boundaries of these three specialties.

A second arena of technologically driven competition has occurred in the treatment of renal disease. Prior to the development of lithotripsy to pulverize renal stones, only surgery, diet, and drug therapy were available (Webb et al., 1986). With the use of lithotripters, radiographic imagery can visualize the renal stones, and sonic waves can break them without surgery. At present, lithotripters are in the urologist's domain and considered part of their technological expertise (Caine, 1986). However, radiologists are beginning to be courted by manufacturers of lithotripters as another market for the machines (Cochran et al., 1987).

These examples serve to demonstrate that the boundaries of medical specialties are not fixed. As medical technology advances, specialists, and subspecialists continue to redefine their domains of expertise. In both examples, at least two separate but related specialties have become direct competitors.

In psychiatry, the treatment of syphilis has undergone a similar shift in specialization. At the turn of the century, syphilis was a prime cause of admission to mental hospitals due to the prevalence of the disease and the limited treatment available for early stages of illness (Solomon and Solomon, 1922). Today, it is a rare phenomenon for a psychiatrist to admit a syphilitic patient. Treatment of syphilis was initially managed by a dermatologist, while the psychiatrist managed the cerebral effects. As pharmacological treatments improved, early treatment of syphilis has become the norm, and it is in the hands of the infectious disease specialist, not the psychiatrist (Brandt, 1985). Ironically, a psychiatrist (Julius Wagner-Jouregg) developed the malarial treatment for certain aspects of the disease and won the Nobel Prize in Medicine and Physiology in 1927. This history of syphilis demonstrates that core medical knowledge and skills are constantly shifting; with these shifts, responsibility for treating patients can and does shift from one specialty to another.

The debates and dialogues that have transpired to push for acceleration of the credentialing process must go beyond an analysis of competition in the marketplace, and who owns the new technology. For psychiatry, we need to determine the boundaries of contemporary psychiatry, and then determine the knowledge and clinical expertise essential to being a competent psychiatrist. Areas of special knowledge or expertise that serve as a basis for subspecialization should be built upon the essential knowledge and clinical expertise of general psychiatry.

Core Knowledge and Expertise in Psychiatry

In the 1980s, the core knowledge and expertise required in psychiatry have been divided into three broad domains. The greatest emphasis is placed on the first two domains, the psychological and the biologic, with social contributions to behavior given less stress. Specific guidelines for teaching core knowledge in residency training programs are determined by the Residency Review Committee (RRC) for Psychiatry, and an accredited residency training program must offer varied clinical experiences in a vast number of patient problems. Included are work with patients having diverse diagnoses, diverse ages, and conditions necessitating varied treatments. Trainees are required to demonstrate varied clinical skills consistent with the patients' needs (Karasu, 1982, 1984). Although the RRC lists a number of core requirements, it is striking that vast differences across residencies in clinical experience and in what is taught or assessed under the same clinical rotation have arisen. And, although the RRC provides a framework, actual implementation of their guidelines is open to interpretation. Operationally, the diversity of residency training experience means there is not an agreed upon core knowledge or experience.

Another example of difficulty in operationalizing the core expertise expected in general psychiatry is presented in the recent APA Task Force on Psychotherapy (Karasu 1982). The report listed modalities of psychotherapy. For training directors, the challenge is to decide which kinds of psychotherapy should be expected of residents training to be psychiatrists. Should we expect every resident to have both clinical experience and supervision in the described 140 psychotherapeutic modalities? Does each resident need to become knowledgeable and proficient in the entire range of psychotherapies? Obviously, providing a full range of clinical experience to meet this hypothetical requirement would be impossible; therefore, what should the core clinical experiences be?

In 1986 and 1987, Weissman and Bashook surveyed senior psychiatric residents to assess the nature of the residents' clinical experiences while in training (unpublished data). When looking at training experiences in long-term psychotherapy (longer than six months) for adults or children across 81 residency programs, there were no consistent patterns of experience shared by a majority of trainees. Without consistent clinical experiences as part of residency training, trainees have no solid background of knowledge and skills and it is very difficult to develop comprehensive fellowship programs on such a shifting foundation. Clearly, there is the necessity of additional training. However, if the knowledge and skills essential to psychiatry have not been defined, where is the boundary between general psychiatry and the subspecialties of psychiatry?

Differences Between Subspecialization in Psychiatry and Internal Medicine

A number of individuals feel that psychiatry should develop credentialing of psychiatric subspecialties following the model of internal medicine. Essentially, they argue that internal medicine has thrived by defining and credentialing subspecialists. The American Board of Internal Medicine accepts the view that a good general internist will have approximately 80 percent of a subspecialist's expertise.

But psychiatry is not internal medicine. The core subspecialties in internal medicine, with two exceptions, are based on organ systems. Each subspecialty focuses on an enhanced understanding of the biologic and pathologic principles that govern a specific organ system. When addressing the cardiovascular system, the subspecialty of cardiology defines the knowledge base and clinical procedures expected of a cardiologist. When the subspecialty is endocrinology, a subspecialty currently without unique procedural skills, the endocrinologist defines the core knowledge base. Clearly, for the specialty of internal medicine, the key organizing principle is the physiology and pathophysiology of a given organ system, or, in the disciplines of infectious disease and oncology, the pathophysiology of a disease process.

There are no obvious equivalent organ systems to understand in psychiatry. Indeed, we have three quite distinct anchors: the biology of behavior and its substrate, the brain; the psychology of behavior, its substrate the brain, and the brain's symbolic creations in affect, language, and behavior; and finally, the influence of environment on our patients and the social and external forces governing behavior. Currently, in studying brain and behavior, there is no consensus on which substances or neurotransmitters to monitor in the blood; we measure only the symbolic communication, as reported in words, or the nonverbal communication, as manifest in affective states.

In contrast, the internist can effectively concentrate on an isolated organ system to focus his or her expertise, to increase the knowledge base, or to improve the value of therapeutic actions. The biological reductionist model of internal medicine would appear ill-suited to address the three separate but related knowledge bases in psychiatry.

Conceptualize Psychiatry Using General Systems Theory

A more appropriate model for organizing psychiatric expertise is contained in the general systems theories developed by Ludwig Von Bertanlanfy (1968), and expanded on by Schwartz and Wiggins (1986). *General systems theory* is the study of an organization and its components in interaction (Encyclopedia Brittanica, 1973). The basic thesis is that complex interrelationships of any type follow similar rules and processes. Because the rules and processes of seemingly unrelated areas are common, it is possible to organize subsystems into larger wholes by understanding the common rules and how they interact with different systems. For example, in psychiatry we would address the interrelations among the various components of our knowledge base in understanding the complex biological factors that affect the syndrome we call *depression*.

In general systems theory, a key rule to developing this interrelationship is the rule of equifinality; a given end result from a complex set of interactions can be obtained from many different initial conditions, by traversing many different pathways (Gedo and Goldberg, 1973). In the treatment of a depressed patient, we know that different treatments may be equally successful, but their success does not imply knowledge of the essential etiology of depression. From a systems theory standpoint, subspecialization based on an arbitrary desire to order data to fit a narrow biologic model will lead, not to advances in psychiatry, but to potentially arrested growth.

A recent example of a narrow reductionistic view is the claim that a biochemical clinical test gave us a biologic marker to diagnose depressions (Carroll, 1980; Carroll et al., 1981). The theoretical model used in this research assumed that depression was a biologic disorder that needed biologic treatment. If it were not for the understanding of behavior brought about by approaching the issue from a general systems theory perspective, we might not have rigorously tested this assumption, and we might not have learned as quickly the limits of the "dex test." The early critique of this test came about because a variety of clinical practitioners, not just psychoneuroendocrinologists, attempted to verify "dex test" results by observing the behavior of their patients (Mullen et al., 1986; American Psychiatric Association, 1987). It is not intuitively obvious that depressed patients have an illness requiring either a biologic, psychologic, or social intervention, or, indeed, any combination of interventions.

This does not, of course, mean that there are not special skills in psychiatry, nor does it mean that each psychiatrist will be expected to be an expert in all of them. For example, the complex behavioral treatment necessary to effectively manage anorexia nervosa patients will not be mastered and need not be mastered by all psychiatrists. However, the existence of special skills or knowledge of eating disorders does not, in and of itself, justify credentialing subspecialists in eating disorders, even though there are specialty journals in this field.

Earlier we noted the ill-defined boundaries for the basics in psychiatry. We must first agree on psychiatry's boundaries and delineate the essential, basic knowledge and skills necessary to general psychiatry. We might then find that advances in current knowledge will lead naturally to the development of subspecialties, which will require formal credentialing.

Psychiatric education will be challenged to avoid developing arbitrary or capricious subspecialty standards based on special interests and to await further maturation of our specialty. Today, we need a plan for postgraduate education that can provide residents and practitioners the necessary core knowledge and clinical expertise and, most importantly, train them to expand their expertise by learning how to continue learning. Those in medical education circles can often be heard urging educators to teach their students how to learn (Green et al., 1984), and urging the teaching of how to learn is an often repeated plea. Self-directed learning, encouraging the development of greater expertise, offers psychiatry an opportunity to develop models, to clarify and enhance the field. The future model of psychiatric subspecialization should evolve, based on the issues unique to psychiatry, from psychiatry, and not as a clone of internal medicine.

The practice of psychiatry is a marriage of three core sciences. This marriage is similar to experiencing an opera. The composer synthesizes orchestral music, vocal music, and drama into a new whole, and it is the unique synthesis of all three artistries that makes a great opera performance. Listening to the "Magic Flute" on a compact disc in one's living room and imagining the drama unfolding on the stage of the Metropolitan Opera in New York is not experiencing an opera performance. In a similar way, understanding and using only neurobiology or psychology for the practice of psychiatry does not make one a psychiatrist. The unique synthesis of all three core sciences in treating a patient is the hallmark of the practice of psychiatry. Anything that detracts from this synthesis is not in the best interest of our profession.

References

American Board of Medical Specialties: Annual Report and Reference Handbook. American Board of Medical Subspecialties, 1987

American Psychiatric Association Task Force on Laboratory Tests in Psychiatry: The dexamethasone suppression test: an overview of its current status in psychiatry. Am J Psychiatry 1987; 144:1253–1262

Brandt AM: No Magic Bullet. New York, Oxford University Press, 1985

Caine M: Contribution of modern lithotripsy to the practice of urology. Isr J Med Sci 1986; 22:237–240

Carroll BJ: Dexamethasone suppression test in depression. Lancet 1980; 1:1249

Carroll B, Feinberg M, Greden F, et al: A specific laboratory test for the diagnosis of melancholia. Arch Gen Psychiatry 1981; 38:15–22

Cochran ST, Barbaric ZL, Mindell HJ, et al: Extracorporeal shock wave lithotripsy: impact on the radiology department of a stone treatment center. Radiology 1987; 163:655–659

Dorros G, Janke LM: Complex coronary angioplasty in patients with prior coronary artery bypass surgery, in situations utilizing multiple coronary angioplasties, and in coronary occlusions. Cardiol Clin 1985; 3:49–71

Encyclopedia Britannica 1966; Vol. 23:281

Flexner A: Medical Education in the United States and Canada (a report to the Carnegie Foundation for the Advancement of Teaching). Bulletin Number 4, Carnegie Foundation, 1910

Gedo JE, Goldberg A: A Model of the Mind: A Psychoanalytic Theory. Chicago, University of Chicago Press, 1973, p 7

Green J, Grosswald SJ, Suter E, et al: Continuing education for the health professions. San Francisco, Jossey-Bass Publishers, 1984

Karasu T: Psychotherapy Research: American Psychiatric Association Commission on Psychotherapies. Washington, DC, American Psychiatric Association, 1982

Karasu T: The Psychiatric Therapies: American Psychiatric Association Commission on Psychiatric Therapies. Washington, DC, American Psychiatric Association, 1984

Ludmerer KM: Learning to Heal. New York, Basic Books, 1985

Mullen P, Linsell C, Parker D: Influence of sleep disturbance and calorie restriction on biological markers for depression. Lancet 1986; 1051–1055

Reeder GS, Vlietstra RE, Mock MB, et al: Comparison of angioplasty and bypass surgery in multivessel coronary artery disease. Int J Cardiol 1986; 10:213–221

Salem BI, Gowda S, Haikal M, et al: Early percutaneous transluminal coronary angioplasty or coronary bypass surgery following thrombolytic treatment of acute myocardial infarction. Chest 1987; 91:648–653

Schwartz MA, Wiggins P: Systems and the structuring of meaning: contributions to a biopsychosocial medicine. Am J Psychiatry 1986; 143:1213

Solomon HC, Solomon MH: Syphilis of the innocent. Washington, DC, United States Interdepartmental Social Hygiene Board, 1922

Von Bertanlanfy L: General Systems Theory. New York, Brazillen, 1968

Webb DR, Payne SR, Wickham JE: Extracorporeal shockwave lithotripsy and percutaneous renal surgery, comparisons, combinations and conclusions. Br J Urol 1986; 58:1–5

Yager J, Langsley D, Peel R, et al: The future psychiatrist as subspecialist: there is no alternative, in Training Psychiatrists for the 90's. Edited by Nadelson C, Robinowitz CB. Washington, DC, American Psychiatric Press, Inc., 1987, pp 129–139

Chapter 4

Subspecialization in Psychiatry

Joel Yager, M.D.

The comedian Jackie Mason tells the story of waking in the middle of the night with pain in his flank, certain that he had a kidney stone. "How," he asked, "do you know who's a good doctor to take care of a kidney stone? Even if your doctor has a diploma on his wall saying that he graduated from medical school with a 90 average, maybe he only got a 60 in kidney!" The average patient is easily as concerned about the physician's technical expertise as about how compassionate and caring the physician is in the doctor–patient relationship. At the same time, concerns that subspecialization and high tech medicine reduce the likelihood that physicians will be wise and compassionate are based partly on the myth that physicians were more compassionate in the "old days." Yet public cynicism about the medical profession over the centuries suggests that physicians have all along had their problems with doctor–patient relationships, whether or not they had technical expertise to bolster their professional reputations.

As we begin to contemplate subspecialization in psychiatry, consider the following questions: first, when colleagues ask for referrals to psychiatrists, how are those requests expressed? In my experience they're often precise: "I need a psychiatrist who can treat an adolescent who's taking cocaine." Or, "I need someone who can handle a manic-depressive with kidney problems taking lithium." Clearly, consumers of psychiatric services, both physicians and the public at large, are increasingly specific in knowing what they need, and they are looking for the best expert advice available. Physicians in disciplines such as internal medicine and surgery, already highly subspecialized fields, have come to expect and demand such special expertise among psychiatrists. A second question: if you or a member of your family were sick, and if there had to be a trade-off between technical expertise and compassion, what would you prefer for yourself, particularly if the problem were serious or enigmatic? A third question: is subspecialization good for us? The answer may depend on who "us" happens to be at the moment: patients, trainees, current practitioners in the community, academics, or organized psychiatry.

The History of Specialization

In 1985 the American Board of Medical Specialties sponsored a conference entitled "Trends in Specialization: Tomorrow's Medicine." The volume resulting from that conference includes an excellent review of this area (Langsley and Darraugh, 1985a). As it happens, the first American specialty organization whose direct descendent ultimately represented a legitimate medical specialty was the Association of Medical Superintendents of American Institutions for the Insane, created in 1844, later to evolve into the American Medical-Psychological Association and then to the American Psychiatric Association. The first medical field to identify itself and to be considered a separate specialty by the medical profession in the United States was ophthalmology in 1861 (Spivey, 1985). This development was directly related to the invention of the ophthalmoscope, and followed the surge in new knowledge about the eye that the instrument provided.

Subspecialization in surgical areas began about 50 years prior to subspecialization in internal medicine, in the first several decades of this century. Surgical procedures lent themselves to a clearer distinction of particular skills. For reasons identical to those currently retarding the development of subspecialties in psychiatry, organized medicine in the United States has periodically instituted moratoriums on the authorization and accreditation of new specialties. In 1972 through 1976, the American Board of Medical Specialties called for such a moratorium, but, like the arms race and perhaps not unrelated psychodynamically, proliferation of subspecialties has been inexorable. Currently there are 23 specialty boards, with a total of over 80 recognized subspecialties. Starting with cardiology in 1941 and with the most recent addition of diagnostic laboratory immunology in 1986, internal medicine now has 12 special certifications. Pediatrics has eight boards, with the recent additions of diagnostic laboratory immunology and pediatric pulmonology in 1986, and pediatric critical care medicine in 1987. Arthur Relman, (1985), editor of the New England Journal of Medicine, projects that, by the end of the decade, 70 percent of physicians will be practicing as specialists even if they are not so certified. And this development is occurring in spite of the pressures of the last two decades to train more primary physicians. Psychiatry currently has only one formal subspecialty board, child psychiatry, but many other areas are emerging as potential subspecialties, including geriatric psychiatry, alcohol and substance abuse, and forensic psychiatry.

Wanting to keep down the proliferation of new specialty boards, the American Board of Medical Specialties, the parent organization, has sought mechanisms for recognizing additional increments of training short of a two-year fellowship experience but consistent with the acquisition of new skills over a 12-month period. Most promising are certificates of *added qualifications,* signifying one year of additional training and contrasting with subspecialty certificates of *special qualifications* that usually signify two or three years of additional training. These mechanisms may be used to recognize certain areas that cross specialties, the so-called *horizontal specialties* such as geriatrics (which crosses internal medicine and family medicine, and perhaps psychiatry), hand surgery (a subspecialty of three different surgical specialties), and critical care medicine (which may be a subspecialty of four to seven primary specialties).

The history of subspecialization is not only progressive but, like evolution, may result in dead ends. A subspecialty may be more likely to find itself defunct or obsolete than a general specialty. *Pthisiology,* pulmonary tuberculous medicine, virtually died with the development of antibiotic treatment for tuberculosis. Similarly, several current specialties and subspecialties may wither as new technologies emerge: for example, the rapid growth of cardiothoracic surgery, in large measure due to the popularity of coronary bypass operations during the past decade, may diminish as these procedures are replaced by angioplasties, which can be performed by cardiologists. Similarly, traditional diagnostic radiology may decline if responsibility for magnetic resonance imaging (MRI) technology ever comes under the control of other medical specialties.

Reasons for Subspecialization

The major impetus for the development of subspecialties, I believe and hope, stems from the rapid advances in science, knowledge, and technology that our profession has enjoyed. These advances have been so profuse that no one person can keep up with all areas of knowledge and skill; and therefore, subspecialty evolution occurs, in professions just as in the rest of biology, as a manifestation of differentiation.

At the same time, students of ethology and sociobiology will easily appreciate the natural tendencies for humans (including physicians) to affiliate in closed groups based on secret initiation rites and esoteric information, fulfilling needs for both clubiness and exclusivity (Tiger, 1969). Sociologically, the esoteric knowledge of subspecialists confers high prestige, because it presumably indicates that they are most competent in a given area. And, in accord with the values of universities, subspecialization has clearly been the road to academic promotion and tenure in medical schools, since during at least the past half decade very few academic department chairs have been appointed who are not subspecialists.

Paul Starr (1982), the prominent medical sociologist, cites competition from outsiders, particularly from non-M.D. specialists, as another major impetus for subspecialty development. Such competition was particularly potent in stimulating the formation of ophthalmology and otolaryngology as separate specialties. Certainly, similar pressures are currently as critical for psychiatry as well, as psychiatrists are now competing with large numbers of nonphysician mental health professionals for patients suffering from alcoholism, substance abuse, family conflicts, and a host of other problems treated with psychotherapy.

Increasing pressures to document individual accountability also add impetus to subspecialization. Hospital privileges now require documentation of increasingly specific skills and credentials. Finally, it has been suggested that subspecialties emerge to remind us where we neglect to adequately train general specialists. In psychiatry, for example, the emerging subspecialties of geriatric psychiatry and alcohol and substance abuse serve to remind us that psychiatry has long neglected these areas in general training programs. They also remind us that we have failed to adequately certify exactly what those trained in general psychiatry are actually competently trained to do.

How Are Subspecialties Created?

The American and Canadian specialties societies have evolved parallel sets of criteria for the establishment of new medical specialties. Sociologically, subspecialties always emerge from the periphery, never from the center of an existing specialty. It is the bold, adventuresome, and innovative academics and practitioners at the fringes of a specialty who establish subspecialties. Specialty or subspecialty recognition is usually sought by a newly formed specialty society supported by strong advocacy leaders in that field within academic institutions. Criteria that have been set forth by credentialing bodies for the recognition of new subspecialties include the following (Darraugh and Langsley, 1985, pp. 21–23):

1. A separate finite core body of knowledge
2. Specific psychomotor activities or skills, for example, certain subspecialized technical procedures
3. Minimum sustaining numbers of subspecialists already practicing de facto
4. The presence of specialty societies and journals (Items 3 and 4 illustrate that subspecialties are formed de jure after they have already formed de facto.)
5. The need for the subspecialty in the community in addition to a desire on the part of teaching hospitals to train in these areas
6. Putative benefits to the health care of the population
7. Consideration of the cost/benefits of establishing the subspecialty (In particular, what are the costs? Will the subspecialty devitalize the parent specialty?)
8. An assessment that the subspecialty is likely to endure, not die out
9. For some fields, identification of a unique affective component, essential in that subspecialty's education, that lends it a separate identity

These criteria are easier to delineate in theory than in practice. Furthermore, many of the various component pieces that lead to the certification of subspecialties have never been demonstrated to have either content or predictive validity. Although it is easy to require that subspecialty fellows obtain specified clinical and educational experiences for a specified length of time, treat a specific number of cases, obtain performance evaluations by supervisors and faculty, and document postfellowship practice requirements, the ultimate assessment of competent terminal behaviors, resulting from such training, through examinations is often more difficult to achieve.

Positive Aspects of Subspecialization

It is generally agreed that subspecialization provides one way to improve the quality of medical practice and education. First, patients can be assured that they are benefiting from the latest in scientific knowledge and technical advances. Second, by concentrating their efforts in one particular area, subspecialty physicians can enhance their expertise and competence and keep their skills at the cutting edge. At the same time, generalists learning from subspecialists can be assured of competent education and consultation. In a study comparing 133 general practitioners with 321 specialists, Rhee and associates (1981) found that when general practitioners practiced without limitation the quality of their care was not as good as that of specialists, and, when the specialists practiced outside their specialty areas, the relative quality of their performances declined.

Subspecialization may also provide protection against malpractice claims. When nonspecialists ask subspecialists to provide second opinions prior to the initiation of a treatment, and the subspecialists indicate that the recommended treatments are appropriate, malpractice judgments are less likely to be awarded.

From a self-serving point of view for practitioners, subspecialization carries economic and prestige advantages. And for researchers, the fact is that research grants are much more likely to be awarded to subspecialists than to generalists. It has even been suggested that, in 10 years, research grants will be awarded primarily to M.D.-Ph.D.s, that is, to those who have clearly subspecialized in research techniques.

The specialty certification process itself also carries benefits. Without certification many who claim to practice a subspecialty or specialty may be unqualified. In World War I, for example, 51 percent of those claiming to be opthalmologists were found by the military to be unqualified (Starr, 1982). Similar concern might be voiced about those who practice psychiatry, although no proof exists one way or the other.

It is also generally felt that pressures for certification improve the standards of training programs. The demands of external certification processes may help training directors, who might otherwise be lax in their evaluations of weak trainees, to adhere to standards. And, because training directors, like deans of medical schools, are not always candid about their graduates and often have a vested interest in portraying them in a sometimes excessively favorable light, external certification processes provide some validation of the adequacy of training. Finally, formal certification procedures provide necessary symbolic rewards for trainees after completion of meaningful educational experiences: the diplomas signify important rites of passage.

Negative Aspects of Subspecialization

With all the aforementioned benefits of formal subspecialization in mind, several thoughtful arguments nevertheless weigh against a headlong rush to subspecialization. In some instances subspecialization may paradoxically reduce the quality of care. If the demand for care is less than the supply of subspecialists, many subspecialists may fail to do enough practice within their subspecialties to maintain proficiency (Spivey, 1985). The danger then also arises that the subspecialists may try to artificially drum up business and do unnecessary procedures. Along these lines, subspecialization may fragment care. If several subspecialists are involved in a case but no one physician assumes responsibility for overall coordination and continuity of care, patients often suffer.

Subspecialization can also add significantly to the cost of care. Subspecialists charge more (and at least thus far insurance companies have complied with differential fees), and the increased length of subspecialty training also increases hospital costs. Moreover, the additional cost of establishing and financing new subspecialty boards is burdensome. No one relishes having to develop and administer more examinations.

Another economic factor is that "base" economic incentives often drive subspecialization. In general, entrepreneurial spirits may oversell the value of subspecialty services, and subspecialists tend to charge as much as the market will bear. However, here psychiatry may demonstrate a somewhat unique development in medical subspecialization. Psychoanalysis can clearly be considered an informal subspecialty of psychiatry, yet many psychoanalysts already charge less per hour for analytic cases than for other cases, simply to assure that they can practice this technique; thus, we now have a situation in which subspecialists may choose to earn less to be able to practice a subspecialty. The same may be true for child psychiatry.

Subspecialization may weaken the core specialty by taking patients and other resources away from general programs by, for example, forcing departments to allocate resources into the creation of new subspecialty services, felt to be necessary primarily to keep up with the competition. In return, strong subspecialty divisions can further fragment core disciplines by initiating efforts to become separate departments, such as departments of child psychiatry. In some European universities, fragmentation into separate academic departments of psychological psychiatry and biological psychiatry has already occurred.

Subspecialization may further fragment the profession as a whole in that physicians may identify first as subspecialists and only second and with the general specialty, as, for example, we have seen with cardiologists and internists. The major parent organizations, such as the American Psychiatric Association, may become less powerful as subspecialists involve themselves more with subspecialty societies like the Academy of Child and Adolescent Psychiatry or the American College of Neuropsychopharmacology.

Academic departments are also susceptible to fragmentation resulting from subspecialization, and, even before general training is completed, medical students, envisioning subspecialty careers, may be further drawn away from comprehensive medical education. They may preoccupy themselves with subspecialty areas far too early in their professional development and neglect some basics.

Weaknesses in the examination process have already been alluded to, particularly those based on cognitive rather than performance measures: to some extent the validity of the certification process remains in question. That is, current assessment methods may inadequately test the extent to which candidates perform competently in actual practice. Improved examination methods are needed for testing both cognitive mastery and clinical competence.

Clear Detriments to Promoting Subspecialties

Here I refer to the multitude of professional problems engendered by subspecialization, as various groups attempt to become more exclusionary. Turf fights are likely to increase in a number of arenas: as gatekeeper systems of care cut down direct access to subspecialists; over the delivery of procedural services, utilization of resources, and marketing; and with respect to who defines competence.

Within departments, subspecialization may result in different tiers of income and privilege, with attendant envy and jealousy. This has already happened in some departments of medicine where procedure-rich subspecialties, such as cardiology and gastroenterology, can demand more of the resources than poorer subspecialties, such as endocrinology.

Disputes over potential restrictions of practice by subspecialty can get particularly ugly. Such disputes could conceivably even be brought to the attention of the Federal Trade Commission, if some groups feel their practices to be unduly restricted. Older psychiatrists, without subspecialty recognition, may feel threatened both narcissistically and economically, by the waves of usually younger and more comprehensively *and* subspecialty trained products of contemporary residency programs.

The Role of the Subspecialist *vis à vis* the General Specialist

In England and Canada, the major and traditional roles of the certified specialists are to consult with primary physicians and, after conducting special diagnostic or therapeutic procedures, to turn care of the patient back to primary physicians. These consultants may also provide ongoing primary care to complex patients. In the United States the situation differs: the large majority of medical subspecialists, and even many surgical subspecialists, practice in their general fields as well as in their subspecialty fields (Aiken et al., 1979). For example, Mendenhall and colleagues' (1979) study found that less than 50 percent of cardiologists' office practices were ordinarily devoted to cardiology consultations and procedures; the rest was spent practicing general internal medicine. Similarly, psychiatrists trained in child psychiatry continue to spend about half their time as generalists seeing adult patients (Marmor, 1975).

In most instances, the well-trained generalist in a specialty can do a large amount of what the subspecialist does. In pulmonary medicine, for example, it has been estimated that general internists can do about 85 to 90 percent of the subspecialty tasks conducted by certified subspecialists (Oliver and Wilson, 1985). Such studies have not yet been conducted for psychiatry; it is known, however, that about half of the psychiatrists who regularly treat adolescents have never taken fellowships in child and adolescent psychiatry (Marmor, 1979). The extent to which such differences in training result in differences to patient outcome has never been assessed.

Concern with the potentially restrictive effects of privileging on practice patterns led the ABMS to adopt the following statement:

> It is recognized that there are various methods for delineating clinical privileges. In making the determination of what privileges a practitioner would be permitted to exercise in a hospital, medical specialty certification or subcertification should be considered as only one of several valid and important criteria. It should be emphasized that there is no specific requirement for a diplomate in a recognized specialty to hold certification in a subspecialty of that field in order to include aspects of that subspecialty within the range of privileges. (Langsley and Darraugh, 1985b, p. 82)

The implications to be drawn for psychiatry are clear: regardless of subspecialization, adequate attention must be given to training general psychiatrists, who, even after subspecialty training, will still be able to provide comprehensive psychiatric care, to subspecialty patients as well as others. To illustrate, substance abuse patients often present with dual, triple, or quadruple psychiatric diagnoses and complex biopsychosocial problem lists that require the care of comprehensively trained psychiatrists, not just narrowly focused subspecialists.

Educational Implications

Subspecialization has influenced general residency training programs in a variety of ways. For example, the field of pediatrics has specified that housestaff rotations to subspecialties should constitute at least 11 but not more than 15 months in a 36-month residency. Neonatology must be scheduled for four to six months, but no more than six months may be spent in any one subspecialty, and the general pediatric residency program must include rotations of at least one month in each of a group of five or six basic subspecialties, with at least eight other subspecialty areas listed as desirable options. As might be expected, within the field of pediatrics significant ongoing disputes occur over which subspecialties should be considered core versus optional subspecialty rotations.

A major advantage of formalized relationships between subspecialties and general residency program is that subspecialty training must be provided to general residents by faculty members who are recognized experts in subspecialty areas and not simply by self-styled experts. By fostering true expertise in faculty, the trend to subspecialization promises to improve the level of training and education in subspecialty areas for all psychiatric housestaff. Such training can occur via subspecialty consultation to general services and/or by housestaff assignment to subspecialty services. In general, psychiatric residency program electives could be devoted to additional subspecialty electives, as already occurs in internal medicine and pediatrics. Alternatively, of course, residents could continue to use their elective time to learn more general psychiatry, equivalent to training in general internal medicine tracks.

Individual training programs will have to attend to their mix of faculty if they are to assure that faculty members competent in each of the emerging subspecialty areas are represented. Even before formal subspecialty certification is available, faculty who are accomplished and active in each of the emerging areas should be included in all training programs, and many programs have already achieved such diversity.

Of course, because not every program will be able to attract all types of faculty members or provide adequate training in all important subspecialty areas, the impetus for regional collaboration and sharing of resources will increase. Such collaborations have already been stimulated by progressively more demanding residency review committee (RRC) requirements.

Can we expect subspecialization to result in an increasing switch in training programs by housestaff as they scamper after various fellowships? Such movement already occurs to some extent. However, it will ultimately be up to each resident program to define whether a resident has successfully completed requirements for general training prior to leaving for a fellowship. Housestaff who train in general residency programs that schedule essential components of training only in postgraduate year four may not be able to switch programs when they reach that level without jeopardizing their status with the American Board of Psychiatry and Neurology. In such situations, the original training-program director may be unwilling to certify to the Board that the houseofficer has successfully completed all the necessary eligibility requirements.

Whole new educational enterprises may evolve to parallel the emergence of subspecialties. Psychiatric educators can be expected to write new volumes of educational goals and objectives, develop new curriculae, and write new subspecialty in-training exams. Parenthetically, it would be of interest to see the extent to which the Psychiatric Resident In-Training Examination (PRITE) and the American Board of Psychiatry and Neurology's written examination can differentiate between those with and those without various subspecialty concentrations or fellowships.

The scarcity of subspecialty trainers, at least in some geographic areas, will require that travelling expert teachers offer courses and consultations at various centers around the country. They must also, then, be available for consultation by telephone, videophone, or electronic network. Inevitably, more training tapes, computer and text-based self-instructional programs, and related learning material will be produced.

To what extent will residency applicants choose general training programs on the basis of the subspecialization options available? Probably to about the same extent as they do now—some, but not much. Those residents who choose large, multi-optioned departments will continue to do so, whereas those who are interested in broad general clinical training, the large majority of applicants, will continue to choose programs by the same criteria they now use.

Other factors will remain important in recruitment: geographic location, program size and emphasis, working conditions, and so on. Increasing numbers of women are now entering psychiatric training, and the influence of this shift on recruitment patterns and on subspecialization is uncertain. Thus, studies are needed to assess whether female applicants give more weight to the geographic requirements of their significant others than do male applicants. With regard to subspecialty training, University of California at Los Angeles (UCLA) female residents have been no less likely than men to take extra fellowships, not only in child psychiatry, and not only by remaining at UCLA for their fellowships. Just as many female residents in internal medicine and pediatrics go on to take subspecialty fellowships, we envision the same development in psychiatry.

We can imagine the following continuum for subspecialty education: Within the four-year general residency, a six-month to one-year "track" can be devoted, as often currently occurs, for subspecialty immersion. Fellowship programs, beginning either in the fourth or fifth postgraduate year after general psychiatry requirements have been met, of one to two years (analogous to child psychiatry) can be established in programs in which appropriate faculty, service, and funding exist. The American Board of Psychiatry and Neurology has recently decided that fellowship programs ultimately leading to certificates of added qualifications will have to begin after the fourth postgraduate year, *after* a full general residency is completed.

Emerging subspecialties will be required to fund not only fellowships, but also national organizations, meetings, journals, and other relevant activities, as described above, all occurring prior to official recognition by the American Board of Medical Specialties. Even without the Board's mechanism, some certification procedures will be established by specialty organizations, as has already occurred for alcohol and drug abuse and for forensic psychiatry. And, as these organizations and their requirements gain legitimacy, their pre-medical specialty *subspecialty* certificates will be seen as increasingly valid.

Subspecialty fellowships will have to be funded by those most interested in a given area. Hospital subspecialty services will fund fellowships from patient revenues. Psychiatric manpower for publicly designated areas of subspecialty need (such as minority, geriatric, or child psychiatry) may still be recruited and funded through programs paid for by the federal government or private foundations. Trainees desiring certain types of additional training may find ways to pay for it themselves, through fees, for example, generated by clinical work. Programs providing subspecialty certificates may be organized through postgraduate university extension divisions, not only for trainees pursuing fellowships immediately after residency training, but also for experienced practitioners wishing to develop subspecialty areas. Such programs will be of particular interest to those who might wish to be "grandfathered" into eligibility for new subspecialty examinations.

One problem that psychiatry can attempt to minimize is that of producing subspecialists who are no longer competent to practice general psychiatry. Although some limitation of practice is to be expected as physicians become progressively specialized, generalist skills should be maintained. By building some continuing general psychiatry experiences into subspecialty fellowship schedules, educators can help preserve the trainees' competence and perspective in general psychiatry.

Finally, subspecialty education and practice may be further upgraded by including other medical specialties, where appropriate, into psychiatry's subspecialty fellowship planning. For example, involving geriatric internal medicine in fundamental components of geriatric psychiatry training, which already occurs in many centers, increases the value of the training. At the Medical College of Virginia, a Division of Alcohol and Substance Abuse has been established with participating faculty from both internal medicine and psychiatry (Lerner et al., 1986). Such crossfertilization may produce a breed of subspecialists able to render better care in their fields than those not receiving such preparation.

Future Issues: The Inevitable

In my view the evolution toward subspecialization in psychiatry is a fait accompli and will continue inexorably. Questions remain as to how we can extract the good of subspecialization while minimizing the problems.

De Facto Licensure

Concern obviously exists that a subspecialty certificate might become a virtual permit or de facto licensure, so how practical would it be for evolving subspecialties to emerge without having to formalize the certification process? Several alternatives can be considered: first, recognition of subspecialization might occur primarily through membership in subspecialty societies that have their own requirements, but this kind of recognition will fall short of formal American Board of Medical Specialties-sponsored certification processes. Second, institution-based subspecialty programs may be accredited by the Accreditation Council on Graduate Medical Education (ACGME), producing de facto subspecialty programs even in the absence of certifying exams for individuals. This mechanism might be suitable, for example, for alcohol and drug abuse or geriatric psychiatry programs. Psychiatrists associated with such programs would presumably be evaluated and monitored under local quality control mechanisms, and their reputations would rise and fall with those of the designated programs. Third, insurance companies and health service-consuming industries might themselves decide to monitor the qualifications of those who claim to provide subspecialty services.

But the question of whether to embrace or reject formal certification for emerging subspecialties remains a central, unresolved problem. Psychiatry will have to observe the natural experiments that will occur and find its own ways.

Resource Allocation

Departments of psychiatry, experiencing pressures to develop several subspecialty areas at once, will have to make strategic decisions about resource allocation. Not all departments will be able to develop all areas, and collaborative regional consortium arrangements may become necessary, even between competing universities. In fact, a University of California at Los Angeles–University of Southern California consortium in geriatrics has already been worked out to provide regional resource sharing. Because many community hospitals will not be able to afford all subspecialists, the potential exists for industrious entrepreneurs to organize subspecialty practice groups that will contract with several community hospitals for services, similar to arrangements that already exist between hospitals and practice groups composed of radiologists and emergency medicine physicians. Through such arrangements, the benefits of subspecialty care can be made increasingly available throughout the community.

Areas of Subspecialization

Psychiatry's currently emerging subspecialties include geriatric psychiatry, alcohol and drug abuse, forensic psychiatry, and psychiatric administration. Other potential areas include psychoanalysis, psychotherapy, family psychiatry, adolescent psychiatry, consultation-liaison psychiatry, psychopharmacology, and hospital-based subspecialties such as ECT. Over the next decade, several new subspecialties may emerge, including those linked to specific disorders (schizophrenia, affective disorders), critical care psychiatry, psychiatric traumatology, computer psychiatry, psychoneuroimmunology (including AIDS psychiatry), nuclear and electronic psychiatry (brain imaging, electroencephalogram-related diagnostics), neurobehavioral psychiatry, and psychiatric molecular genetics. While some of these are likely to remain academic center-based subspecialties, they are not idle fantasies. Indeed, a number of recent psychiatric graduates have entered nuclear-imaging fellowships in several programs across the country. Most are interested in research, but they also foresee developing practice areas with these techniques.

Like other fields of medicine, psychiatry will no doubt develop both *academic specialties* and *practice specialties,* as Paul Beeson (1980) has called them. Beeson defines academic specialties as those heavily research-oriented areas forced to remain within universities, primarily because they aren't able to generate an economically viable practice base in the community. Practice specialties are those which best succeed when chronic diseases are involved: they include good basic science correlations, complex diagnostic technologies performed by the specialist, a variety of palliative measures, the lack of a simple and curative treatment, a large volume of literature being produced, and available third party payment. Geriatric psychiatry and substance abuse appear to be evolving in this direction.

Realistic Recruitment Goals

As psychiatry begins to anticipate subspecialization, the field may be able to attempt some rational manpower planning. How well can we estimate how many psychiatric subspecialists of each type the country needs? The Graduate Medical Education National Advisory Council (GMENAC) has already estimated needs for child psychiatry. A newer national group, the Council on Graduate Medical Education (COGME), will continue to study manpower needs. The national societies of geriatric psychiatrists, alcohol and drug abuse specialties, and other groups may also find it useful to develop similar projections, on which national policies for subspecialty fellowship planning can be based. Perhaps we can avoid the traps evident elsewhere in medicine of overproducing physicians who may be underutilized in their subspecialty areas. To the extent that psychoanalysis represents a psychiatric subspecialty, overproduction with respect to the demands for practice of this subspecialty may have already occurred (not that the psychoanalytic training per se has been without value for psychodynamically informed psychotherapy). Many trained psychoanalysts often do relatively little pure psychoanalytic practice, due as much to the lack of suitable paying patients as to other factors. The excessive production of subspecialists elsewhere in medicine has led to what Robert Chase (1976, p. 497) has called "mandatory overqualification for the task at hand." But we can rest assured: this state of affairs does not yet exist in psychiatry.

References

Aiken LH, Lewis CE, Craig J, et al: The contribution of specialists to the delivery of primary care: a new perspective. N Engl J Med 1979; 300:1363–1370

Beeson P: The national history of medical subspecialties. Ann Intern Med 1980; 93:624–626

Chase RA: Proliferation of certification in medical specialties: productive or counter productive? N Engl J Med 1976; 294:497–499

Darraugh JH, Langsley DG: Certification of medical specialists in the United States and Canada, in Trends in Specialization: Tomorrow's Medicine. Edited by Langsley DG, Darraugh JH. Evanston, IL, American Board of Medical Specialties, 1985, pp 1–25

Langsley DG, Darraugh JH (eds): Trends in specialization: Tomorrow's Medicine. Evanston, IL, American Board of Medical Specialties, 1985, pp. 1–97(a), pp 77–86(b)

Lerner WD, Forbes RO, Merlin SI, et al: A division of substance abuse medicine in a teaching hospital. Journal of Medical Education 1986; 61:606–608

Marmor J: Psychiatrists and Their Patients. Washington, DC: Joint Information Service of the American Psychiatric Association and the National Association of Mental Health, 1975, p 20

Mendenhall RC, Tarbor AR, Givard RA, et al: A national survey of internal medicine and its specialties: II. primary care in internal medicine. Ann Intern Med 1979; 91:275–287

Oliver TK Jr, Wilson DR: Economics of subspecialty education and certification, in Trends in Specialization: Tomorrow's Medicine. Edited by Langsley DG, Darraugh JH. Evanston, IL, American Board of Medical Specialties, 1985, pp 65–66

Relman AS: Meeting tomorrow's manpower needs: how do we get from here to there?, in Trends in Specialization: Tomorrow's Medicine. Edited by Langsley DG, Darraugh JH. Evanston, IL, American Board of Medical Specialties, 1985, pp 53–57

Rhee S, Luke RD, Lyons TF, et al: Domaine of practice and the quality of physician performance. Med Care 1981; 19:14–23

Spivey BE: Today's health care system: the role of specialization in the United States, in Trends in Specialization: Tomorrow's Medicine. Edited by Langsley DG, Darraugh JH. Evanston, IL, American Board of Medical Specialties, 1985, pp 27–42

Starr P: The Social Transformation of American Medicine. New York, Basic Books, 1982

Tiger L: Men in Groups. New York, Vintage Books, 1969

Chapter 5

The Future of Consultation– Liaison Psychiatry as a Psychiatric Subspecialty

Jeffrey L. Houpt, M.D.

Currently there are significant concerns about the economics of health care and the implications for psychiatry in general. As fiscal intermediaries search for ways to economize, one needs to be concerned about the proportion of the total health care dollar that will be assigned to psychiatry. Consultation activities in particular are vulnerable, because they have historically been underreimbursed. Liaison activities have traditionally required funding independent of patient care.

In addition, there are concerns within the field about subspecialization as has been outlined in Chapter 4 in this book. There are concerns about fractionalizing the field, and whether psychiatry can maintain a coherent identity. Consultation–liaison psychiatry finds itself a logical choice for consideration as a subspecialty and thus finds itself drawn to the center of this controversy. Consequently the subject of the future of consultation–liaison psychiatry has important meaning for the field in general, as well as for that specific field dedicated to consultation and liaison activities. This chapter addresses issues and concerns about the economics of health care and subspecialization. The first section considers definitions of the areas under inquiry; the second section puts forward assumptions underlying the predictions; next, predictions on the future of consultation–liaison psychiatry are considered; and finally, the implications of this reasoning are outlined.

Definitions

For purposes of this chapter, *consultation–liaison psychiatry* is defined as that activity wherein psychiatric knowledge and skills are applied to patients located within the general health care sector. Traditionally, two specific functions have been identified: consultation—providing advice about patient diagnosis or treatment; and liaison—teaching about the biopsychosocial interactions relevant to patient care. In neither instance does the psychiatrist routinely take primary responsibility for patient care.

Increasingly, however, the psychiatrist has been assuming primary responsibility for patients in the general health sector with combined medical and psychiatric morbidity. For the purposes of this paper, *psychiatric medicine,* or *medical psychiatry,* is the term designated to refer to that area in which the psychiatrist assumes primary responsibility for the diagnosis and treatment of patients with both medical and psychiatric disorders; the internist (or other specialist) becomes the consultant and follows the patient in a secondary capacity.

These activities can take place in any segment of the general health sector—an outpatient primary care setting, a community hospital, or a tertiary care referral hospital. Thus, the field of activity of the psychiatrist to be covered in this chapter will be viewed in terms of responsibility to the patient (consultation to the primary physician, teaching to the health care team, direct patient responsibility) and setting (primary care outpatient, community hospital, tertiary referral hospital). This is depicted in Figure 1.

This grid will be used as a stimulus for considering the future of consultation–liaison psychiatry, after considering the assumptions on which this argument is based.

Assumptions

Assumption I

The most basic assumption of this chapter is that the American public will continue to believe that 10 percent to 11 percent of the gross national product is sufficient for health care, and that employers will continue to look for ways of selling their goods least expensively and thus continue to limit the

		Primary Care Out-patient	Community Hospital	Tertiary Referral Hospital
PSYCHIATRIST ACTIVITY	Consultation			
	Liaison			
	Primary patient responsibility			

Figure 1.   General health sector

amount health care contributes to the cost of their product. Buicks will compete better with Toyotas if General Motors can decrease health care costs. As a result, even greater emphasis will be placed on providing efficient, effective, and inexpensive care. Presently the most intriguing means for keeping psychiatric costs in line appear to be capitated services and managed care companies. Capitated systems limit the amount of money available per person or provider, whereas managed care companies review all procedures and, in effect, manage a person's access to services. Whether or not these systems prove to be effective is yet to be fully tested. However, some form of cost control can be anticipated. Based on this assumption, the following conclusions can be drawn.

Traditional consultation–liaison functions will not be able to fund themselves. History suggests that consultation–liaison psychiatry requires external funding to thrive. Consultation–liaison psychiatry can trace its present-day form to a series of grants in the 1930s and 1940s from the Rockefeller Foundation to Harvard University (Massachusetts General Hospital), the University of Colorado, the University of Chicago, Tulane University, Washington University in St. Louis, and Duke University. All received grants to begin consultation–liaison divisions. The goal was to bring psychiatry into the medical setting, making its diagnostic and therapeutic functions available to medical patients. A variety of models to deliver patient care and teaching developed, not only at these institutions but others as well.

After a period of excitement, interest in the field dwindled until renewed interest was stimulated by the Psychiatry Education Branch of the National Institute of Mental Health (NIMH) in the 1970s. Just as the first thrust of consultation–liaison psychiatry depended on Rockefeller Foundation funds, so its second thrust required external funding. Consultation–liaison services experienced a major period of growth in the 1970s, through grants from the Psychiatry Education Branch of NIMH. These grants were competitive, were reviewed by study sections, and required site visits in their earliest years. Competition pushed these programs to seriously evaluate themselves, which in turn resulted in their incorporating educational methods and technologies. With the withdrawal of NIMH funding in the 1980s, however, the size of consultation–liaison programs decreased.

Because direct patient care provides its own funding, psychiatric medicine will emerge as a cost-effective and popular alternative. Psychiatrists specializing in medical and psychiatric comorbidity should prove popular to managed care companies. They should be able to provide more effective, and perhaps even more cost-effective, treatment than the internist with psychiatric consultation. Likewise, in a capitated system, medically oriented psychiatrists might well excel, because they are skilled in taking care of very sick patients. Referring physicians prefer that the psychiatrist take care of the psychiatrically impaired, so long as the medical condition can be managed through their consultation, and thus psychiatric medicine should be popular with the internist or surgeon as well.

Level of care distinctions will become sharper.   More patients will be held in the outpatient sector, community hospitals will care for the more routine patient, and tertiary care hospitals will receive patients who are sicker, have multiple diagnoses, or need high technology treatment.

As a consequence of the economic climate, greater attention will be paid to the intensity of care, and the placement of the patient in the most appropriate and least costly setting. There will be disincentives to moving the patient into hospitals, and patients who are admitted to hospitals will thus be sicker. Fiscal intermediaries will increasingly insist that community hospitals receive the "routine," less complicated patients: gall bladder, hysterectomies, fractures, routine gynecology, and so forth. Tertiary care hospitals will receive complicated patients, often with multiple diagnoses. This will include the elderly with depression and with disease of several organ systems.

Tertiary care hospitals will increasingly resemble 600-bed intensive care units. Only the very sick, or those who require the latest high tech care, such as transplant patients, will be admitted. In all these instances, aberrant behavior, psychiatric disorder, and stress within the delivery system will encourage psychiatric attention, but in the form of the psychiatrist taking a more hands-on approach than traditional consultation.

Assumption II

Our second assumption holds that changing demographics will result in a larger demented population. Census Bureau projections call for increases in the two aging populations—those over 65 and those over 85—with a 20 percent increase in the over-65 age group and an 88 percent increase in those over 85, by the year 2000. This compares with an estimated 7 percent to 10 percent increase in the overall general population. As the prevalence of dementia is estimated at 3 percent of those aged 65 and over and at 20 percent of those over the age of 80, one can easily infer a significant increase in demented patients within our hospitals.

In addition, we can expect increases in a younger group of patients with dementia due to the acquired immune deficiency syndrome (AIDS). Some health planners predict that, without a successful treatment for AIDS, a majority of beds will be occupied by these patients in some hospitals, particularly in urban areas. Approximately 30 percent to 40 percent of AIDS patients show signs and symptoms of central nervous system (CNS) dysfunction, and 80 percent show postmortem neuropathological abnormalities that are generally associated with neuropsychiatric symptoms. In short, both of these groups will increase the requirement for psychiatric diagnostic and therapeutic skills in the general hospital.

Assumption III

The third assumption holds that the scientific knowledge base will continue to grow, and, along with economic conditions, will force subspecialization. For example, just 10 years ago, it was sufficient to know that tricyclic antidepressants should be used cautiously in patients with cardiac disease. The psychiatrist was advised to obtain an ECG in patients over 40, and to obtain a cardiology consultation routinely in patients with an abnormal ECG. We now know significantly more about the effects of cyclic antidepressants and, as a result, modern standards require significantly more monitoring. The psychiatrist working in medical settings is now expected to evaluate many diverse factors: which patients with first degree or second degree block are at risk; what ECG monitoring is required; whether left bundle branch block, left anterior fasicular block, or right bundle branch block represent significant cardiac pathology.

Similarly, standards of knowledge have changed significantly in the area of organic brain syndromes. Discussions of 10 years ago were limited to diagnosing delerium or dementia. Skills in the mental status exam, brief neuropsychological screening exams, and knowledge of the role of the EEG or CAT scan defined the competent psychiatrist; the ability to diagnose the specific etiology was not considered necessary. Today, that has changed. Now it is necessary to know and to work up the most frequent causes for delerium and dementia. Neurologic consultation is often requested when interpreting results or evaluating uncommon cases, rather than to merely suggest what tests to order routinely. This trend of increased primary responsibility for care and increased knowledge base will continue into the future.

Predictions

Our predictions for the future of consultation–liaison psychiatry follow from the aforegoing assumptions. These best-guess estimates are formulated according to the grid developed earlier. A summary of these predictions is shown in Figure 2.

		Primary Care Out-patient	Community Hospital	Tertiary Referral Hospital
PSYCHIATRIST ACTIVITY	Consultation	Little to none	Same for psychiatrist, increase for psychologist	Subspecialists
	Liaison	Mental health professionals other than psychiatrist	Virtually none	Virtually none
	Primary patient responsibility	MSW uncomplicated	Behavioral medicine; transfer to psychiatrist	Med/psych units; ancillary behavioral med labs and neuropsychology

Figure 2. General health sector

Within the Primary Care/Outpatient General Health Sector

Consultation.   This sector will continue to grow in size and will attempt to retain patients not referred to hospitals to try to control costs. Casefinding will be a function of the primary care physician, and there will be virtually no psychiatric consultation in this setting.

Liaison.   As teaching, liaison will continue as long as family practice programs and primary care internal medicine programs continue, and teaching efforts within specialty-oriented internal medicine programs will decrease to virtually zero. The present trend toward using mental health professionals other than psychiatrists as teachers will continue, making liaison activities by psychiatrists in these settings rare, if at all existent.

Direct patient responsibility.   This will continue to grow as capitated systems grow. As has been true of health maintenance organizations, patients will be referred to the lowest cost therapist. Social workers have nearly replaced psychologists in some of the larger health maintenance organizations, and we can expect this trend to continue, as well as the use of master's level counselors. Patients referred for psychotherapy will be seen in groups or in time-limited psychotherapies. Patients treated in these programs will have relatively uncomplicated problems. Those with more complicated problems— combined medical-psychiatric disorders or psychiatric disorders such as severe depressions, borderline personality disorders, bipolar disorder, and schizophrenia—will get little to no definitive treatment within the primary care/outpatient general health sector. Some may receive referrals, as they do presently or, alternatively, patients may "force" treatment by requiring inpatient care. They will be admitted to general hospitals with combined medical-psychiatric problems or to psychiatric units, either free-standing or within general hospitals, with psychiatric problems without medical complications. A large public mental health system will continue to exist, in effect, to take patients removed from the private sector.

Within the General Community Hospital

Consultation.   The time-honored tradition of consultation will continue. It will not undergo a resurgence but rather will continue much as in its present mode. Depressed, suicidal, psychotic, somatosizing, and drug-abusing patients will continue to be referred. This level of consultation requires no additional training and will be done by general psychiatrists.

Psychologists will assume a larger role in some settings, either where there are too few psychiatrists or where they offer something distinctly different from psychiatrists. This would include behavioral medicine services or neuropsychological evaluation. The application of behavioral approaches to medical patients will likely remain a core skill of the psychologist and only occasionally will psychiatrists have these skills. Both behavioral medicine, including biofeedback labs, and formal psychodiagnostic evaluations, especially neuropsychological assessment, will provide psychologists their entry into the general health care sector, and they will then share the psychotherapy referrals as a result.

Liaison. As a teaching function, virtually none will take place. Psychiatrists will be guest speakers at the monthly medical staff meeting, on occasion. There will be no formal teaching programs.

Direct patient responsibilities. We will likely see the growth of behavioral medicine laboratories, with direct patient care falling within that context. General psychiatrists will continue to transfer patients from the general hospital medical service to psychiatric services to the consulting psychiatrist's choice of free-standing psychiatric hospital, or to his or her office for treatment. By and large, these referred patients will suffer from primary psychiatric disorders, with minimal medical overlay.

Within the Tertiary Care Hospital

Consultation. Consultation will continue to be provided primarily by the psychiatrist, with some additional assistance from psychologists. Psychiatrists will take the lead because patients will have comorbidity (medical and psychiatric). The proper dissection and integration of biopsychosocial components of these patients' care will require a psychiatrist. He or she may request neuropsychological or behavioral intervention, but the complexity of the cases will require the integrating abilities of a physician.

However, in distinction to the community hospital, the consultation within tertiary care centers will be done by a subspecialist, a *medical psychiatrist*. Because these cases will be the most complicated cases with comorbidity, a generalist will not be sufficient.

Liaison. Liaison teaching will be minimal to nearly nonexistent. Formal teaching programs for medical housestaff will not exist. A medical psychiatrist with the time and inclination might pause to discuss a case, as internists might do now with psychiatric professionals. There may be some conjoint medicine/psychiatry or surgery/psychiatry meetings, as, for example, oncology or transplant surgery might sponsor an ongoing case review. However, the identity of the medical psychiatrist will be that of a care giver, not a consultant or teacher. Both of these latter activities will be incidental to the major task of getting the appropriate patient to his or her service for treatment.

Direct patient responsibility. Medical psychiatry units will become common in nearly all tertiary care university hospitals. They will exist to treat that group of people with combined medical and psychiatric problems, who have been held on medical units with psychiatric consultation in the past.

The medical psychiatric unit is, and will remain, a sound fiscal alternative to traditional consultation and liaison activities. Reimbursement from inpatient charges will remain much more secure than consultative fees. Even with Medicare reimbursement rates, as many patients will be geriatric patients, inpatient work will be more stable financially because of the efficiency and volume of service. Behavioral physiology labs will be commonplace. They will form the financial base for behavioral medicine units, and will be an adjunctive treatment for some patients, and a primary treatment for others.

With all of this "medicalization," what will become of the psychotherapists among us? Medical psychiatrists will continue to use brief psychotherapy and family interventions. Their success will depend in part on being skilled in those areas. If the psychiatrist is not personally skilled, he or she will have to delegate it to another member of the health care team. Without psychotherapeutic skills, the medical psychiatrist will not be able to successfully or efficiently treat these patients. Further, these skills, and their use in shortening hospital stays, will further delineate psychotherapists from the behaviorally oriented neurologist.

Implications

This scenario would predict that psychiatric medicine will become a subspecialty of psychiatry. It differs significantly from consultation–liaison psychiatry, as it is practiced at this time.

Distinct from consultation–liaison psychiatry, psychiatric medicine is specifically concerned with the care of patients with combined medical and psychiatric disorders. Providing advice or teaching are not valued to the same degree as in consultation–liaison psychiatry. Routine consultations as they are done now do not and probably will not require subspecialization. General psychiatrists will continue to carry out this function.

Psychiatric medicine requires a much deeper knowledge base. It is not enough to know the phenomenology of dementia, delerium, or organic affective syndrome; the new medical psychiatrist knows how to work up the major conditions causing these disorders. The medical psychiatrist will use other specialists as consultants to his or her practice. Specialists will help interpret work-ups, provide advice for treating the medical disorder, or suggest alternative etiologies when appropriate.

Medical psychiatrists will need to become more expert in pharmacology, particularly as it relates to medical illness and drug–drug interactions. Rather than securing a medical consultation for patients with combined morbidity who need psychotropic medication, the medical psychiatrist may recommend psychotropic agents in the medically ill because of his or her special knowledge of the pharmacologic actions and side-effects of the psychotropic agent. A thorough understanding of cardiac-conduction difficulties and an ability to read an ECG will be required. The ability to think through a medical problem, such as selecting the proper cyclic antidepressant for a patient with myasthenia gravis, will be required.

The medical psychiatrist will need to retain skills in the physical exam. Morning hospital rounds will find the psychiatrist listening to lungs, to abdomens for bowel sounds, repeating the neurologic exam, examining for bed sores, and so forth. The medical psychiatrist will clearly do the physical exam on admission.

More than likely there will be significant debate on how one is best trained for this position. Should one be "double-boarded" to medicine and psychiatry, or triple-boarded as in pediatrics, psychiatry, and child psychiatry? This debate will continue to rage, just as it did earlier in consultation–liaison psychiatry, when the question was whether one had to have training in medicine to be effective as a consultation–liaison teacher. The answer for medical psychiatry will probably be the same: Many good, competent medical psychiatrists will have traditional psychiatric training, whereas others will have more than one year of medical training, and double-boarding will not be required. Fellowship programs will likely include more neurology and medicine, and this will be good for the profession.

It is important to emphasize that these psychiatrists will not be "junior internists." The medical psychiatrist will continue to maintain a primary identity as a psychiatrist; he or she will require expert medical consultation. What is shifting here is the location of the patient—from medicine to psychiatry beds—and the focus of primary patient care responsibility—from the internist (or other specialist) to the psychiatrist.

Finding the proper name for this speciality is important. *Psychiatric medicine* or *medical psychiatry* will be doomed for failure, as it should be, if it implies that the rest of psychiatry is nonmedical. *Consultation–liaison psychiatry,* as a name for this field, has the advantage of being known, but it also has the problem of an implied secondary, rather than primary, care role. In addition, it refers to a process or delivery system model, rather than a discrete body of knowledge. It may be that reformulation of the term consultation–liaison, and consistent subsequent usage, will solve these problems, but consideration should be given to other terms for this field as well. Whatever the term, it needs to imply primary patient responsibility, a growing subspecialized field with greater emphasis on the knowledge base, and a decreased emphasis on teaching other specialists to treat psychiatric disorders.

In short, I propose that consultation–liaison psychiatry, defined as patient consultation and teaching, is a transitional stage while we move toward the medical psychiatrist. These current functions of the consultation–liaison psychiatrist will remain within the realm of general psychiatry, but those psychiatrists who take primary responsibility for the medically and psychiatrically ill will emerge as subspecialists in psychiatric medicine or consultation–liaison psychiatry as a reformulated term and field.

Chapter 6

The Future of Addiction Medicine as a Psychiatric Subspecialty

Marc Galanter, M.D.
Zebulon Taintor, M.D.

Alcohol and Drug Abuse: The Historical Context

The medical profession has been slow in recognizing alcoholism and drug abuse as legitimate medical illnesses. In large part, this is the result of the social forces which have influenced treatment of these syndromes, forces which have operated to define the nature of illness at other times in history. It is characteristic of the care of the infirm that certain sick people are labeled as morally defective and undesirable, rather than as suffering from legitimate diseases. This was well illustrated by Foucault (1973) in his assessment of Western European attitudes toward the mentally ill. He noted that after leprosy had virtually disappeared from Europe in the early 17th century and leprosaria had been closed, attitudes toward the psychologically disturbed and behaviorally deviant began to change. If there were no lepers to be seen as unacceptable, another group of infirm had to be thrust into that role. Over several decades, asylums and "ships of fools" were established to assure the isolation of these unfortunates, who had previously been allowed to mingle freely among the general population. As time went on, these mentally ill were treated with increasing harshness. It was only some two centuries later, with the advent of "moral treatment" for mental illness, that humane attitudes toward the mentally ill were widely applied in Europe.

The labeling of the rejected, with their consequent inhumane treatment, can also be seen in American attitudes toward addicted persons. This took place after the use of opiates came to be associated with the oriental laborers, a socially rejected group, of the Pacific Northwest in the late 19th century. Similarly, the chronic, socially debilitated alcoholic came to occupy a rejected role until the mid-20th century, and the person with alcoholism was presumed to be morally afflicted. It is therefore understandable that these social attitudes would serve to define the scope of medical attention (and thus education) in the addictions, as well as for our view of the addicted person.

57

Little attention was paid to the proper mode of rehabilitation of the addicted patient, and failure to improve was thought to be related to moral turpitude.

Over recent decades, however, our country has begun to deal less judgmentally with the issues of alcoholism and drug abuse. In 1935, because of the absence of available, competent, medical care for alcoholism, people with alcoholism banded together to form Alcoholics Anonymous (AA). This organization, which now has a membership of more than 1.5 million people worldwide, adopted as one of its early tenets the notion of alcoholism as a disease. The emergence of Alcoholics Anonymous has had an important effect on American attitudes. Alcoholics Anonymous demonstrated that the alcoholic person could regain a constructive place in society and was therefore not beyond reclaim. It also showed that the recovered alcoholic, an upright citizen, was not a tainted or incompetent person.

In the field of drug abuse, social connotations associated with criminality and lower social class also led physicians to turn away from an active treatment and rehabilitation role. The heroin epidemic of the late 1960s and the consequent attempts to find a large-scale solution led to federal initiatives that resulted in nearly 100,000 Americans being placed in methadone maintenance treatment programs. The prescription of methadone and attention to psychiatric and rehabilitative aspects of treatment led to a greater medical focus on opiate addiction. This coalesced with the establishment of the National Institute on Drug Abuse (as well as the National Institute on Alcohol Abuse and Alcoholism) in 1973 and a rapid growth of research into underlying biological, psychological, and social mechanisms of addiction. The institutes, in turn, fostered the training of physicians as career teachers, and thus subspecialists of a sort were born.

What changes are now coming about in physicians' attitudes toward alcohol and drug abuse? It is well documented that alcohol and drug abuse are etiologic and precipitating factors in a large portion of medical illness. One hospital survey indicated that one-fifth of male medical inpatients are alcoholics, and, for most of these patients, alcohol was a primary precipitant of their illness (Barcha et al., 1968). In psychiatric services, substance abuse was found to be a major factor involved in two-fifths of inpatient admissions (Crowley et al., 1974) and one-half of emergency room visits (Atkinson, 1973).

Despite these findings, the clinical importance of substance abuse had long been underplayed in medical education until recent years. This largely reflected physicians' attitudes toward the addictions as issues holding only a secondary place in their disciplines. The American Medical Association, however, through its Council on Mental Health, issued a position paper in 1972 on the importance of placing greater emphasis on drug and alcohol abuse in medical education (Galanter, 1980). It emphasized that medical educators' efforts should be directed at correcting prevailing stereotypes, and that students should be sensitized to the physician's function as a gatekeeper to available drugs for the abuse. A literature on professional training in alcoholism and drug abuse was beginning to develop, derived both from national conferences (Seixas and Sutton, 1971) and from actual medical school curricula (Stimmel, 1974).

In this context, the federal government in 1971 undertook planning of a program that would support medical school faculty members interested in teaching in substance abuse. Designated as *career teachers* in alcohol and drug abuse, these faculty were to be supported by federal grants for a period of three years. Upon the establishment of the National Institute on Alcohol Abuse and Alcoholism and the National Institute on Drug Abuse, the career teacher program was undertaken as a joint endeavor by the new institutes. Altogether, career teachers were funded in 59 medical schools under this program, which came to an end in 1983. Importantly, the career teachers collaborated with the National Board of Medical Examiners to formulate questions on substance abuse for the national boards.

To assure continuation of their work, the career teacher group established the Association for Medical Education and Research in Substance Abuse. This group, initially synonymous with the career teachers group itself, has served as the nucleus for augmenting the course of substance-abuse training, research, and treatment on medical campuses throughout the country. The Association now has a membership of over 400.

Subspecialization in Addiction Medicine

The path to subspecialization in this area does not proceed from a specialty to a subspecialty, as has happened with forensic psychiatry, but from various specialties, as has happened with child psychiatry's entry from either psychiatry or pediatrics. This can be understood by the need to work back from the sequelae of substance abuse. Initially, substance abuse was viewed as a medical problem only in relation to its sequelae. Physicians were involved according to whatever specialty treated particular sequelae best: internal medicine for cirrhosis of the liver, psychiatry for alcohol-related psychoses, and so forth.

Can anything regarding specialty involvement be learned from Alcoholics Anonymous' conceptualization of alcoholism as a disease? That concept would seem to dictate medical intervention, but help was provided by one's peers rather than physicians. Physicians suspected that Alcoholics Anonymous was antimedical, and the relationship with psychiatry was complicated by an injunction to members to avoid mood-altering medicines, lest they again become dependent. Alcoholics Anonymous members complained that physicians were unresponsive.

In 1954, the American Medical Association declared alcoholism to be a medical illness and called for more attention to this ubiquitous problem, but it did not take a position on which specialty(ies) should pay such attention. Rather, each physician was to decide involvement based on personal interest. Shortly thereafter, a society was formed by physicians concerned with alcoholism treatment, and by 1982 the group had a membership of over 800. Today, under the name of the American Medical Society on Alcoholism and

Other Drug Dependencies, the organization has a membership of 2800 and certifies physicians for their expertise in this field. Membership in this group is largely nonpsychiatric, with psychiatrists constituting only 34 percent (Galanter et al., 1983). No other specialty dominates.

The issue of subspecialty certification moved forward dramatically in 1985 when the Society's certification process was established. In 1986, the first examinations were given; by 1987, 1250 physicians had been certified, but only 28 percent of those applying to take the examination were psychiatrists. In psychiatry, on the other hand, the American Academy of Psychiatrists in Alcoholism and the Addictions was established in 1985, growing to a membership of about 800 within two years. It has established a center for. medical fellowships in alcoholism and drug abuse at New York University School of Medicine and began to define preliminary criteria for fellowship training in the field.

The American Psychiatric Association Study on Psychiatric Education

This study was conducted by the American Psychiatric Association to ascertain the current status in America of psychiatric education in alcoholism and drug abuse. It was done in conjunction with similar surveys in general internal medicine, pediatrics, and family practice training programs. Altogether, 106 of 124 medical school departments of psychiatry and 169 of 220 psychiatric residency programs responded. Of the respondents, 97 percent of undergraduate and 91 percent of residency programs offered curriculum units in alcoholism and drug abuse, and certification units in the large majority of both undergraduate and residency programs were required. Most programs also provided a training context, with supervised clinical care. Nonetheless, certain areas of dissatisfaction were reported, among them, attitude and interest of faculty and curriculum time allotted. The committee conducting the study concluded that there appeared to be a growing amount of time allotted to alcoholism and drug abuse curriculum, but the quality of teaching commitment was still in question. Because of this, further investment in developing faculty fellowships in addiction was seen to be warranted.

American Academy of Psychiatrists in Alcoholism and the Addictions Survey of Current Fellowship Programs

In 1987, the 211 psychiatry residencies in the United States were circularized by the Education Committee of the American Academy of Psychiatrists in Alcoholism and the Addictions and the Center for Postgraduate Training in Alcoholism and Drug Abuse at New York University School of Medicine for information on fellowships in substance abuse (Galanter, 1987). The results were heartening in that there were more programs established than had been previously realized. Of the 124 residencies who responded (59 percent of the sample), 20 reported having fellowships, 34 reported being interested in establishing fellowships, and 69 reported no interest. Fifteen of the 29 fellowship programs had begun after 1984, and, at the time of the survey, 29 fellows were enrolled in these programs. Half of the programs had one or two students, another five had three or four, and five programs did not currently have any enrollees. Programs generally required a completed residency, and were open to nonpsychiatrists. (Only eight were restricted to psychiatrists.) Most (85%) required completion of four or more years of postgraduate training (PGY 4) prior to acceptance.

In terms of duration of fellowship, 80 percent required at least one year; 65 percent offered more than one year. The alcohol and drug abuse components were evenly balanced (50%–50% or 60%–40%) in most of the programs. Training emphasis differed among the programs, but 12 allotted at least 50 percent to clinical time. Fifteen programs allotted at least 10 percent to teaching others (for example, medical students). Seven allocated at least 20 percent of the fellows' time to research.

Why Addiction Medicine Should Be a Subspecialty of Psychiatry

There are many approaches that could be taken in answering this question. Historically, psychiatry has been the most involved of the medical specialties, granted that there could have been more involvement, and that psychiatry's involvement was offset by prominent individual members of other specialties. Psychiatry is the only medical specialty to have given increasing prominence to the substance abuse treatment experience in its special requirements for an approved residency program.

The reasons that psychiatry has been involved in the past are arguments for its continued and greater involvement: it is involved with the psychological and sociocultural dimensions of its patients in a way that other specialties are not. Ingesting a potentially harmful substance *voluntarily* involves an element of free will. The social contexts of alcoholism and drug abuse/dependency, themselves different from one another, also influence outcome, to a degree not found in most medical illnesses. Psychiatry, as the specialty that pays special attention to synthesizing its treatment plans by integrating across the multiple frames of reference that make up the biological, psychological, and social dimensions of its patients, is best equipped to foster a subspecialty in addiction medicine. The proposed core curriculum illustrates the argument.

Core Curriculum for Substance Abuse Subspecialties

The American Psychiatric Association's study proposed minimum knowledge, skill, and attitude levels for medical students, residents, and continuing education are given in the appendix. For the purposes of this discussion, it is important to note that a different end point is proposed for each general category. The medical student level is essentially the same as what would be expected of any nonpsychiatric physician; continuing education for nonpsychiatric physicians is not considered and will doubtlessly vary (as will continuing education for psychiatrists) as the field changes. To the different levels of knowledge and skills in the appendix are added suggestions for fellows (below). These are requirements expected of subspecialists. Attitudes were not specified according to educational level, although willingness to engage and the other attitudes set forth in the appendix are crucial to good patient care and have determined much of the history of the field thus far.

The Future of Fellowships

There is a considerable need for training of medical specialists in alcoholism and drug abuse. The magnitude of the substance abuse problem today is well documented, with the cost to the public calculated at over $150 billion per year in health care and lost work. Furthermore, as noted above, a large portion of general medical patients present with substance abuse problems, many of which go undiagnosed. When the sequelae of addiction, such as cirrhosis, trauma, and infection, are present, they often receive medical attention, while the patients' primary addictive problems themselves go untreated. Clearly, training has been inadequate to date. Compounding this problem is the fact that federal support for medical education in substance abuse has been curtailed in the last five years, in that the federal Career Teacher Program, which had successfully supported faculty in five medical schools during the previous decade was terminated in 1982.

As the substance abuse field matures, it is essential that the principal trainees in medical teaching centers—medical students and residents—be exposed to properly trained faculty, who can serve as role models in the mainstream of medical care. To achieve this end, a procedure for fellowship training within the academic model is necessary for developing a cadre of educators and researchers.

The legitimacy of medical subspecialties and their ability to establish standards of training and attract trainees has traditionally rested on various forms of the board certification process. The likely option for such training is a certificate of added qualification, defined in Chapter 3. This current procedure of the American Board of Medical Specialties entails modification of specialty certification to reflect that a candidate has completed at least one year of full-time formal training in a subspecialty program and has passed an additional examination prepared by a member board. Geriatric medicine was the first such program to be established, in 1987. This process can be instituted by any of the medical specialties, to institutionalize post-residency training in alcoholism and drug abuse and promote development of a cadre of physicians who will serve as medical teachers for the field. It is with this eventual goal of formal certification in mind that fellowship training standards for the substance abuse field can be established, as proposed here by the Education Committee of the American Academy of Psychiatrists of Alcoholism and Addictions in collaboration with the Association for Medical Education and Research in Substance Abuse.

The following guidelines were prepared by the Education Committee of the American Academy of Psychiatrists in Alcoholism and Addictions (Galanter, 1987), as a working model for persons establishing fellowships:

The purpose of substance abuse postgraduate medical fellowships is to 1) assure high quality care; 2) provide teaching and research faculty at medical centers; and 3) define clinical and academic standards for the field. Such fellowships will contribute to the development of the medical field of substance abuse, much like fellowships in specialty areas, such as cardiology or pediatric endocrinology, in earlier decades.

The American Board of Medical Specialties' standard relevant here is that specialty certifications with added qualifications (see Chapter 3) can be developed under the American Board of Medical Specialties, with at least one year additional training and an examination. The American Board of Internal Medicine, for example, instituted such a procedure for geriatrics.

Certain components of *training* in an additional fellowship are agreed on by leading figures in field:

1. Relevant basic science training in each of these areas: biochemistry, pharmacology, epidemiology, social theories, genetic models, behavioral conditioning models
2. Supervised clinical experience in each of these areas:
   a. settings: inpatient and outpatient
   b. drugs: alcohol, opiates, and other drugs of abuse
   c. clinical laboratory testing
   d. therapies: pharmacotherapy; individual, group, and family therapy, self-help; consultation, team leadership; detoxification and rehabilitation
   e. special problems: including dual psychiatric and addictive illness, adolescents
3. Research: participation in ongoing research and/or an original project related to addictive illness
4. Education: teaching medical students, house staff, and other personnel

Place in the Training Sequence

A two-year experience is preferred, either 1) a postgraduate year 5, if there has been previous specialized experience; 2) postgraduate years 4 and 5; or 3) postgraduate years 5 and 6.

Conclusions

The arguments for addiction medicine as a psychiatric subspecialty are:

1. The clinical need is enormous and well documented.
2. Levels of attainment for medical students, nonpsychiatric physicians, psychiatric residents, continuing education for psychiatrists, and fellows have

been thought through and found, through a national survey, to be in place in many programs.

3. Although different specialties have been involved in the past as a result of treating alcoholism and drug abuse sequelae, psychiatry is most relevant in terms of the knowledge and skill base it has to offer.
4. Subspecialty fellowships have evolved.
5. Subspecialization is proceeding through self-designated certification by the American Medical Society on Alcoholism and Other Drug Dependencies and examinations through the American Academy of Psychiatrists in Alcoholism and the Addictions.
6. The drive toward subspecialization should now be channeled and regulated.

References

Atkinson RM: Importance of alcohol and drug abuse in psychiatric emergencies. Calif Med 1973; 118:1–4

Barcha R, Stewart MA, Guze SB: The prevalence of alcoholism among general hospital ward patients. Am J Psychiatry 1968; 125:133–136

Crowley TJ, Chesluk D, Dilts S, et al: Drug and alcohol abuse among psychiatric admissions. Arch Gen Psychiatry 1974; 30:13–20

Foucault M: Madness and Civilization. New York, Vintage Books, 1973

Galanter M: The career teacher program, in Alcohol and Drug Abuse in Medical Education. Edited by Galanter M. Washington, DC, U.S. Government Printing Office, 1980, 20–26

Galanter M: Postgraduate medical fellowships in alcoholism and drug abuse. New York, American Academy of Psychiatrists in Alcoholism and Addictions, 1987

Galanter M, Blume S, Bissell L: Physicians in alcoholism: a study of current status and future needs. Alcoholism Clin Exper Res 1983; 7: 389–392

Seixas FA, Sutton JY (eds): Professional training on alcoholism. Ann NY Acad Sci 1971; 178:1–139

Stimmel B: The development of a curriculum in drug dependency. Med Educ 1974; 49:158–162

APPENDIX

Minimum Knowledge and Skill Levels in Addiction Medicine

The American Psychiatric Association study proposed the following minimum knowledge and skill levels of alcohol and other drug use curricula in psychiatry for the different levels of professional with which medical educators deal: medical students, residents, and practitioners taking continuing education.

Continuing education requirements are as of 1987. In general, medical student objectives are in the form of skills.

1. **General Concepts in Addiction Medicine**

   - **Alcohol and other drug use/abuse: biopsychosocial context**
     Medical Students
     Should have a broad knowledge of biopsychosocial model, intellectual understanding of how substance abuse fits in
     Residents
     Should be able to apply biopsychosocial model and fit substance into it
     Practitioners/Continuing Education
     Should master the idea of biopsychosocial models

   - **Disease concept of drug use/abuse**
     Medical Students
     Should understand why substance abuse is a disease rather than merely a moral or social problem
     Residents
     Should be able to teach others the concept of substance abuse
     Practitioners/Continuing Education
     Should be able to fit substance abuse in with other psychiatric diagnoses

   - **Definition of dependence**
     Medical Students
     Should know the definitions of use, abuse, dependence, addiction
     Residents
     Should be able to apply the definitions of use, abuse, dependence, addiction
     Practitioners/Continuing Education
     Should be able to apply the definitions of use, abuse, dependence, addiction

   - **Natural history and etiology**
     Medical Students
     Should have broad knowledge of parallels to other chronic illnesses, role of free will, peer group issues

Residents

Should have detailed knowledge of range of outcomes for specific substances, patient types, psychological variables

Practitioners/Continuing Education

Should know natural history and etiology of more recently introduced substances of abuse (e.g., crack, angel dust, MDMA, etc.)

2. Basic Sciences

- **Pharmacology: receptors, reinforcement, tolerance, dependence; human pharmacology, pharmacokinetics, drug interactions**

  Medical Students

  Should be able to relate substance abuse to pharmacology course

  Residents

  Should master clinical applications of psychopharmacology of drugs of abuse and relate to commonly used psychoactive medications

  Practitioners/Continuing Education

  Should know clinical applications of recent psychopharmacological finding of drugs of abuse

- **Neurochemistry and neurophysiology**

  Medical Students

  Should be able to relate substance abuse to neurochemistry and neurophysiology courses

  Residents

  Should demonstrate the actions of drugs of abuse in relationship to principal neurochemical and neurophysiological mechanisms

  Practitioners/Continuing Education

  Should introduce recent findings in neurochemistry and neurophysiology as they relate to clinical management of substance abusers

- **Toxicology**

  Medical Students

  Should be able to place toxicology of abused substances in the context of other toxins studied

  Residents

  Should master the toxicities of drugs of abuse, counsel pregnant patients

  Practitioners/Continuing Education

  Should know recent findings related to substance abuse toxicology (e.g., cardiotoxicity of high doses of cocaine)

- **Genetics: population genetics**

  Medical Students

  Should learn substance abuse population genetics as part of a general course

Residents

> Should have expert knowledge of population genetics and ability to do genetic counseling

Practitioners/Continuing Education

> Should introduce recent findings in genetics of substance abuse (e.g., transmissibility of drug addiction)

- **Genetics: molecular genetics**

Medical Students

> Should be aware of molecular underpinnings of genetic vulnerabilities

Residents

> Should know genetic influences of metabolism and addiction vulnerabilities of different species (e.g., mice)

Practitioners/Continuing Education

> Should introduce recent findings in molecular bases of genetic vulnerability

- **Behavioral sciences: behavioral psychology**

Medical Students

> Should be introduced to concepts of reinforcement and conditioning and their relation to addiction

Residents

> Should show how behavioral principles apply to specific clinical aspects of addiction and rehabilitation

Practitioners/Continuing Education

> Should introduce recent findings in behavioral psychology (e.g., physiological correlates of conditioning)

- **Behavioral sciences: psychodynamics**

Medical Students

> Should know basic psychodynamic mechanisms mediating experimentation, use, abuse, and dependency

Residents

> Should be able to teach psychodynamic mechanisms

Practitioners/Continuing Education

> Should know recent contributions to psychodynamic theory

- **Behavioral sciences: family systems**

Medical Students

> Should know basic mechanisms

Residents

> Should be able to draw upon sociocultural factors in formulating a case

Practitioners/Continuing Education

> Should be aware of recent developments in use related to sociocultural factors

3. **Epidemiology and Demography**

- **Incidence and prevalence among various demographic groups**
  Medical Students
  Should know how surveys are performed and possible sources of bias; should have an idea of recent trends
  Residents
  Should be able to design a survey, know recent findings and implications for treatment and service provision
  Practitioners/Continuing Education
  Should know recent survey data

- **Risk factors**
  Medical Students
  Should be aware of concept of risk factors and how these are derived
  Residents
  Should be able to use knowledge of major risk factors in case formulation
  Practitioners/Continuing Education
  Should know recent risk-factor findings

4. **Prevention**

- **Avoidance of iatrogenic disorders: managing chronic pain**
  Medical Students
  Should be aware of how management of chronic pain can produce iatrogenic problems
  Residents
  Should know alternate means of managing chronic pain
  Practitioners/Continuing Education
  Should know recently introduced analgesics and techniques

- **Recognition of high-risk populations, situations, lifestyles**
  Medical Students
  Should know populations, common features of such situations and lifestyles
  Residents
  Should know well enough to teach medical students
  Practitioners/Continuing Education
  Should be aware of recent developments

- **Community health resources, health promotion**
  Medical Students
  Should know types of resources available and how to use them
  Residents
  Should know national and local resources; be able to design a program
  Practitioners/Continuing Education
  Should have experience participating in prevention exercises

5. Medical Assessment: Comprehensive Historical and Physical Evaluation

- **Alcohol and other drug history**
  Medical Students
  Should be able to record use
  Residents
  Should understand and interpret denial and underreporting
  Practitioners/Continuing Education
  Should know typical use patterns of newly developed drugs

- **Family history: psychiatric illness, alcohol/other drug abuse**
  Medical Students
  Should be able to obtain historical facts
  Residents
  Should be able to construct family trees of use
  Practitioners/Continuing Education
  Should be aware of how recent genetic research findings are expressed in family use/abuse patterns

- **Other medical and psychiatric histories**
  Medical Students
  Should be able to perform basic review of systems
  Residents
  Should be able to integrate review of systems into biopsychosocial formulation
  Practitioners/Continuing Education
  Should be aware of recent developments in history taking

- **Physical examination**
  Medical Students
  Should be able to detect moderate/severe substance abuse
  Residents
  Should be able to detect mild/minimal substance abuse
  Practitioners/Continuing Education
  Should be aware of physical findings of recently fashionable drugs

- **Prior alcohol and other drug abuse treatment**
  Medical Students
  Should have knowledge of types of treatment
  Residents
  Should be able to assess whether treatment was appropriate: assess interplay of patient and treatment variables to explain outcome
  Practitioners/Continuing Education
  Should have knowledge of new forms of treatment

- **Mental status examination**
  Medical Students
  Should be able to perform basic mental status exam

Residents
Should be able to interpret subtle findings
Practitioners/Continuing Education
Should be aware of findings for recently developed drugs

- **Interpretation of laboratory tests**
Medical Students
Should have knowledge of what basic tests can be abnormal
Residents
Should have experience interpreting wide range of test findings, false-positives, etc.
Practitioners/Continuing Education
Should have knowledge of recently developed tests

- **Personal, social, and economic histories**
Medical Students
Should have general awareness of economics of substance abuse and effects on interpersonal relationships
Residents
Should have knowledge of economic, personal, and social factors connected with wide variety of specific drugs
Practitioners/Continuing Education
Should have knowledge of such factors related to recent drugs

- **Appropriate use of consultants**
Medical Students
Should have knowledge of consultation resources
Residents
Should be able to use consultants, serve as consultant
Practitioners/Continuing Education
Should be aware of need for consultation related to recent drugs

6. **Diagnosis and Differential Diagnosis**

- **Diagnosis of alcohol/other drug disorders**
Medical Students
Should have knowledge of main factors to be used in making a differential diagnosis
Residents
Should have practice making differential diagnoses in 50 cases
Practitioners/Continuing Education
Should be aware of differential diagnostic problems posed by recent drugs

- **Multiple diagnoses: coexisting medical/psychiatric conditions**
Medical Students
Should understand concepts of comorbidity and causality
Residents
Should have experience in how multiple diagnoses can affect treatment

Practitioners/Continuing Education
Should be aware of increasing incidence of multiple diagnoses

- **DSM and ICD diagnostic criteria**
  Medical Students
  Should know definitions
  Residents
  Should have experience in 50 cases of use of diagnostic criteria
  Practitioners/Continuing Education
  Should be aware of recently developed diagnostic schema

- **Individualized formulation and treatment plans**
  Medical Students
  Should have knowledge of typical goals and objectives for substance abuse treatment
  Residents
  Should have written goals and objectives for 50 cases: be able to lead multidisciplinary treatment team discussions
  Practitioners/Continuing Education
  Should be aware of treatment planning for new clinical problems

7. **Intervention, Confrontation, and Referral**

- **Intervention/confrontation techniques: evaluate potential for harm to self and others**
  Medical Students
  Should be aware of common signs of lethality
  Residents
  Should be able to apply the literature on risks in 50 cases
  Practitioners/Continuing Education
  Should be aware of potentials posed by recent drugs

- **Intervention/confrontation techniques: establish a therapeutic alliance**
  Medical Students
  Should be able to perform initial interviews, counsel
  Residents
  Should be able to establish a psychotherapeutic relationship in most motivated cases
  Practitioners/Continuing Education
  Should be aware of therapeutic alliance problems associated with recent drugs

- **Intervention/confrontation techniques: motivate patient for treatment and recovery**
  Medical Students
  Should have knowledge of factors leading to enhanced motivation
  Residents
  Should have experience increasing motivation in 10 patients

Practitioners/Continuing Education

Should be aware of motivational issues posed by recent drugs

- **Intervention/confrontation techniques: intervention strategies with family and network**

  Medical Students

  Should have knowledge of how family and social networks can be used

  Residents

  Should have experience using family and social networks in 10 patients

  Practitioners/Continuing Education

  Should be aware of family and network issues posed by new drugs

- **Referral resources: community resources/agencies**

  Medical Students

  Should have knowledge of community agencies to which referrals can be made

  Residents

  Should have used community resources in 10 cases

  Practitioners/Continuing Education

  Should be aware of new agencies and the services they offer

- **Referral resources: self-help groups**

  Medical Students

  Should be aware of special roles of various self-help groups

  Residents

  Should have experience using self-help groups; have attended some meetings; know relationship between mode of action and other treatment

  Practitioners/Continuing Education

  Should be aware of new groups

- **Referral procedures: knowledge of referral**

  Medical Students

  Should know some referral resources

  Residents

  Should be aware of many referral resources

  Practitioners/Continuing Education

  Should be aware of any new procedures

- **Referral procedures: effecting the referral**

  Medical Students

  Should know how to refer

  Residents

  Should have referred successfully in 10 cases

  Practitioners/Continuing Education

  Should be aware of any new methods

- **Referral procedures: follow up the referral**
  Medical Students
     Should know how to follow up
  Residents
     Should have successfully followed up 10 cases
  Practitioners/Continuing Education
     Should be aware of any new follow up procedures (e.g., confidentiality changes)

8. **Other Medical and Psychiatric Complications**

   - **Effects of alcohol/other drugs on fetus and newborn**
     Medical Students
        Should know general effects
     Residents
        Should be able to integrate specific pathophysiological mechanisms
     Practitioners/Continuing Education
        Should be aware of recent research findings

   - **Trauma**
     Medical Students
        Should know general effects
     Residents
        Should have treated cases in which trauma was a complication
     Practitioners/Continuing Education
        Should be aware of recent research findings

   - **Chronic pathology associated with the toxic effects of alcohol/other drugs**
     Medical Students
        Should know effects
     Residents
        Should have treated patients with alcoholism and cirrhosis
     Practitioners/Continuing Education
        Should be aware of chronic pathology associated with new drugs

   - **Medical consequences of routes of administration**
     Medical Students
        Should know consequences of various routes
     Residents
        Should have treated heroin addicts with infections
     Practitioners/Continuing Education
        Should be aware of recent drug complications (e.g., cocaine and the nose)

   - **Dangerousness and violence assessment**
     Medical Students
        Should be aware of methodology

Residents
Should have carried out 20 assessments
Practitioners/Continuing Education
Should be aware of complications of new drugs

- **Influence on family, work, and social functioning**
Medical Students
Should be aware of influences
Residents
Should have helped 10 patients work with these issues
Practitioners/Continuing Education
Should be aware of effects of recent drugs

9. **Acute and Long-Term Management**

- **Acute management: intoxication**
Medical Students
Should know basic management mechanisms
Residents
Should have managed 10 cases of intoxication
Practitioners/Continuing Education
Should be aware of intoxication management issues for recent drugs

- **Acute management: withdrawal**
Medical Students
Should know basic management issues
Residents
Should have managed withdrawal in 10 cases
Practitioners/Continuing Education
Should know withdrawal course for recent drugs

- **Acute management: overdose**
Medical Students
Should know how to manage overdose
Residents
Should have managed overdose in 10 cases
Practitioners/Continuing Education
Should know how to manage recent drugs

- **Long-term management: establish long-term relationships**
Medical Students
Should know how such relationships are established
Residents
Should have established 5 such relationships
Practitioners/Continuing Education
Should know of recent developments in establishing such relationships (social changes, personality variables associated with new drugs)

- **Long-term management: treatment modalities and expected outcomes**
  Medical Students
  Should know modalities and expected outcomes
  Residents
  Should be able to use various modalities
  Practitioners/Continuing Education
  Should know new modalities and findings on efficacy

- **Long-term management: pharmacotherapy of primary alcohol/ other drug abuse conditions**
  Medical Students
  Should know medications used
  Residents
  Should have used medications in 10 cases
  Practitioners/Continuing Education
  Should know recently developed medications

- **Long-term management: pharmacotherapy of other/associated medical or psychiatric conditions**
  Medical Students
  Should know medications used
  Residents
  Should have used medication in 10 cases
  Practitioners/Continuing Education
  Should know recently developed medications

- **Long-term management: participation in an interdisciplinary team**
  Medical Students
  Should have experience in a clerkship
  Residents
  Should have led a team for treatment of 10 cases
  Practitioners/Continuing Education
  Should know of recent team developments

10. Legal Aspects

- **Knowledge of DEA schedule of controlled substances**
  Medical Students
  Should know schedule groups
  Residents
  Should know drugs on schedule
  Practitioners/Continuing Education
  Should know recent drugs added to schedule

- **Screening tests: blood, urine, breathalyzer, saliva, etc.**
  Medical Students
  Should know tests

Residents
   Should have used tests and can interpret results
Practitioners/Continuing Education
   Should know recently developed tests

- **Criminal and civil liabilities associated with alcohol/other drugs**
  Medical Students
     Should know liabilities
  Residents
     Should have helped patients deal with liabilities
  Practitioners/Continuing Education
     Should know recent changes in liabilities (e.g., decriminalization, victim rights)

- **Patient privacy, confidentiality, dangerousness**
  Medical Students
     Should know patient rights versus others rights
  Residents
     Should have experienced these issues in treating 10 cases
  Practitioners/Continuing Education
     Should be aware of recent developments

Attitudes Important to Addiction Medicine

Attitudes are considered separately from knowledge and skills because they bear on all of the previous issues.

- **A fresh look at old problems**
  Medical Students
     Should know the issues in maintaining this attitude
  Residents
     Should have this interpreted in supervision
  Practitioners/Continuing Education
     Should experience exercises designed to elicit and rejuvenate attitudes

- **A willingness to examine one's professional style**
  Medical Students
     Should initiate professional style, be aware of method to examine
  Residents
     Should be able to develop style
  Practitioners/Continuing Education
     Should be able to reexamine developed style

- **Revision of old stereotypes**
  Medical Students
     Should be aware of how stereotypes develop and can be revised

Residents

Should have his/her stereotypes elicited and modified in supervision

Practitioners/Continuing Education

Should revise stereotypes by incorporating new knowledge

- **Realism about alcohol/other drug abuse as a chronic disease**
Medical Students

  Should appreciate issue from education

  Residents

  Should incorporate by providing treatment

  Practitioners/Continuing Education

  Should maintain by keeping abreast of research

- **Appropriate optimism about individual patient's potential**
Medical Students

  Should be aware of tendency to be overly pessimistic

  Residents

  Should develop by providing treatment

  Practitioners/Continuing Education

  Should maintain through new knowledge

- **Ability to recognize the disease in a patient or professional colleague**
Medical Students

  Should be aware of data on physicians/other professionals who are impaired

  Residents

  Should have abilities verified through supervision

  Practitioners/Continuing Education

  Should have involvement in impaired-physician presentations or groups

Chapter 7

The Future of Psychiatric Education

Jerald Kay, M.D.
Alan Tasman, M.D.

As David Rogers recently warned, "A sudden deluge of new developments promises to change medicine and medical practice more swiftly than at any time in the past, and some of the possible developments have the potential for making medicine less than it should be, with unfortunate consequences for both physicians and the larger society" (Rogers, 1985, p. 2404). Numerous articles have appeared recently in important journals decrying new restraints on the practice and organization of medicine (Relman, 1987; Berrien, 1987; Alper, 1987; Kralewski et al., 1987) and the need for reassessing the overall image of medicine (Beeson, 1987). Indeed a sign of the times may have been the convening of a recent joint American Medical Association, Association of American Medical Colleges, and American Hospital Association conference entitled "The Medical Profession: Enduring Values and New Challenges." The purpose of this conference was to explore how the medical profession can retain and extend its historic social role as a learned profession, in an era of rapidly increasing biomedical knowledge and effectively applied technology, when there is competitive commercialization of medical care and restricted resources for its support (Association of American Medical Colleges, 1987b).

These issues speak to important forces affecting medical education and highlight the fact that medical training will continue to be unquestionably and inextricably tied to the nation's economy and to new patterns of health care delivery. The implications of this are already evident in the economic forces that constrain the academic health sciences center, after a long period of limitless growth and expansion (Ginsberg, 1984). All of the new forces impinging on the training of physicians will need to be understood if we are to intelligently and optimistically plan for the future of psychiatric education. Only then can we make use of the exciting potential of the rapidly expanding scientific psychiatric knowledge base.

The Educational Milieu

Economics

In 1987, health care costs represented 11.2 percent of the gross national product (GNP) and are likely to account for 15 percent of the GNP by the year 2000. It is understandable, therefore, that health care costs have become a major policy concern and cost-containment efforts are now so prominent. A major component of these efforts has been a variety of prospective payment plans for Medicare and other forms of health insurance. State governments have been moving toward tighter restrictions for eligibility and coverage of Medicaid services. Industry has made consistent and increasing copayments and deductibles a part of its cost-containment efforts. These have been accompanied by shifting allegiances to less expensive health plans through health maintenance organizations, independent practice associations (IPAs) and prospective payment organizations, corporate contracts, and the increasing use of gatekeeping through employee assistance programs (EAPs). A recent survey of 293 companies indicated that more than half are using one or more methods to manage inpatient mental health care costs of their employees (More Companies Manage Health Care Costs, 1988, p. 18). These methods included precertification, concurrent review, data analysis, case management, and retrospective review. Nearly half sponsored an EAP, and nearly two-thirds tracked use of their mental health plans since 1983.

All of these cost-containment measures are coming at a time of increasing need for medical and psychiatric treatment, especially with respect to the chronically mentally ill, the elderly, the unemployed, those with acquired immunodeficiency syndrome (AIDS), and the major impact of the coming of age of the baby boom population and its attendant increase in young adulthood mental illness.

New Characteristics of Care Delivery

Psychiatric care delivery, shaped by economic, demographic, and epidemiologic forces, also has undergone significant change over the last quarter century. With the anticipated surplus of physicians by 1990, the importance of primary care physicians in the delivery of mental health services grows. Currently, more than half of all Americans with mental disorders are treated in the primary care and general health sector, and only 15 percent are seen by mental health specialists (Regier et al., 1978). Deinstitutionalization has profoundly challenged the structure and delivery of mental health services too.

In recent times, private psychiatric office practice has changed considerably, with fewer psychiatrists working exclusively in this setting. Corporate, institutional, and managed group practices continue to grow, as private practice becomes endangered through more stringent competition and regulation. Competition between psychiatrists and other mental health specialists has intensified as the numbers of psychologists and social workers has tripled since 1955 (Goldman and Ridgely, in press). Cost containment, the oversupply of physicians, and competition between mental health providers will provide persistent economic threats to the delivery of services by psychiatrists and could genuinely threaten the job satisfaction and economic rewards of the private practice of psychiatry. Training programs will need to consider the changing practice patterns much more than in the past when designing curricula.

Financing Psychiatric Training and Education

All of the new forces impinging on the current and future practice of medicine in general, and of psychiatry in particular, will affect the future of undergraduate and graduate psychiatric education. The most potent of forces, however, are the economic ones. The funding mechanisms for residency training in psychiatry, as in all of medicine, are under attack. Traditionally, residency training has been supported through cross-subsidization via pass-throughs factored into daily hospital charges, use of Medicare Part B billing, and a host of related mechanisms that provided for resident stipends and fringe benefits, as well as for faculty and other indirect costs. As more than 80 percent of the funding for residency training comes from Blue Cross, other commercial insurance, Medicare, Medicaid, and hospital appropriations (Association of American Medical Colleges, 1985), the shift from a retrospective to a prospective reimbursement system has produced a crisis in the financing of graduate medical education (Schwartz et al., 1985; Relman, 1984). Moreover, federal support for indirect costs has declined dramatically since 1985. When costs for patient care, therefore, are calculated to include teaching costs not found in nonteaching community hospitals, hospitals no longer receive total reimbursement. Not only are urban teaching hospitals reported to have substantially higher operating costs, but they also provide caring for indigent and sicker patients with more complex medical problems (United States Department of Health and Human Services, 1986). Indeed, in 1981, the average per-case cost for the 115 largest teaching hospitals was $3705, compared to $1698 for the average nonteaching hospital (The Commonwealth Fund, 1985). Reimbursement patterns from Medicare and Medicaid also complicate training programs, by emphasizing decreased patient lengths of stay and promoting practices of "dumping" less desirable patients (Schiff et al., 1986). New models for additional funding of graduate medical education include: 1) requiring residents to pay tuition for training; 2) taxing all health care to provide training reimbursement to teaching institutions (Petersdorf, 1985); 3) developing payback arrangements between institutions and residents; 4) linking care for the indigent to training cost reimbursement (Rieselbach and Jackson, 1986); 5) working without compensation; and 6) permitting residents to work under supervision in community settings while being paid for their services.

Reimbursement problems and competition between academic medical centers and community- and investor-owned hospitals have placed increasing demands on faculty to generate their own salaries with potential endangerment of clinical research and educational excellence (Guggenheim and Nadelson, 1984; Kay, 1987a). Cost-containment efforts through prospective payment have also introduced important questions about training experiences conducted under strict length-of-stay regulations. These include issues of limitation of certain treatments, the restriction of patient populations by diagnosis and severity of illness, and possibly higher patient mortality rates (Shortell and Hughes, 1988).

The most recent controversial issue, which has profound economic implications for financing graduate medical education, has been that of resident working hours and supervision. In response to the Zion case in New York City (Asch and Parker 1988), a number of recommendations from organized medicine have been made regarding the need for graduate physician supervision of residents in critical care areas, as well as restricting the number of hours a house officer may work, including those devoted to moonlighting activities. While it has been advocated that teaching hospitals be reimbursed by health care payers for extra costs that might be incurred if residents' workloads are reduced, there have been no systematic plans for such. Resident welfare and wellbeing issues are likely to remain prominent and will require both economic and curricular adjustments to residency training programs.

Changing Clinical Settings

Practice settings in psychiatry are evolving rapidly and challenge the training programs to provide residents with attitudes, skills, and knowledge equally applicable in a multiplicity of care systems. Prospective payment systems have spawned many new forms of organized care settings, including health maintenance organizations, prospective payment organizations, and IPAs, all demanding new practice styles and raising important training issues. Should residency training focus on general skills that can be applied to all settings or should specific skills for each setting be taught? Because of an emphasis on brief or time-limited interventions, new settings may also jeopardize optimal experiences in continuity of care and long-term psychotherapeutic treatment relationships. A related and critical problem concerns the viability of clinical research in new settings that are guided strongly by economic objectives. Further, cost-containment efforts and changing clinical settings of care delivery have brought a new focus to the role of ambulatory care teaching in undergraduate and graduate medical education (Association of American Medical Colleges, 1986a).

The Chronically Mentally Ill

Deinstitutionalization has permitted the discharge of massive numbers of state hospital patients over the last 10 years. There is great concern, however, that many of these patients have never been integrated into community-based care, and now constitute a new class of patients (Goldman et al., 1983). Both this failure to provide for former state hospital patients and the development of a new group of young, chronically ill, adult patients, will affect training experiences. These patients frequently have complex medical and psychiatric conditions that require leadership and treatment skills that only psychiatrists, by virtue of their training, can provide. Because the increased availability of mental health service provided by nonpsychiatrists will have selected impact on this group, future psychiatrists will have to be trained to meet the clinical and administrative needs of the chronically mentally ill largely in the public sector.

New Research and Technology

Recent developments in neurobiology, epidemiology, psychopharmacology, treatment assessment, and psychosocial and environmental factors in the pathogenesis of physical and mental disorders have made psychiatry more scientific. New areas under investigation include neurotransmitter and receptor mapping, an expanded understanding of the mechanisms of action of pharmacological agents, brain-imaging techniques, the elucidation of genetic patterns for major mental illness, the ability through longitudinal studies to identify at-risk populations early in life, increased understanding of mechanisms and treatment for diseases like Alzheimer's disease, useful psychotherapeutic outcome and efficacy studies, an appreciation of the psychosocial contributions to physical illness, and the delineation of mechanisms and treatments for substance abuse (Nadelson and Robinowitz, 1987).

The challenge facing psychiatry, and psychiatric training programs in particular, is not only to integrate this scientific explosion in practice and education, but to prepare future practitioners for a professional lifetime of such growth. Residency training must address fundamental questions in defining basic and specialized skills appropriate for the future practice of psychiatry. Some of these questions include the following: 1) What is the role of subspecialization? 2) What constitutes a core curriculum for all residents? 3) How much training is required in specialty areas like child and geriatric psychiatry? 4) What should be the role of psychotherapy training? 5) Should research experiences be required and how should they be taught? 6) How should continuing self-education be promoted? Answers to these and other questions are of central importance to the design of the new residency training curriculum. In addition to predicting future practice models, the training director will need to struggle with presenting trainees with a reasonably well-balanced and inclusive program, during a time of increasing service systems demands and funding tensions.

Recruitment

Data collected in the 1970s and early 1980s by medical and education organizations indicated a dramatic decline in the number of American medical students entering the field of psychiatry. This occurred even while the specialty was predicted by the Graduate Medical Education National Advisory Council (GMENAC) to have the greatest shortage. In 1968, the Health Resources Administration reported that 12 percent of American medical graduates entered psychiatric residencies. By 1980, however, the National Residency Matching Program (NRMP) was noting that 2.7 percent of United States medical school seniors did so. A national conference on psychiatric manpower and recruitment was convened in 1980 to discuss this problem. Specific recommendations regarding new strategies to enhance recruitment were developed and assigned to appropriate psychiatric organizations for implementation. Recommendations addressed the need for greater visibility of psychiatry at the college and medical school level through more rigorous teaching, greater socialization, better rewards for student teaching, active and unambivalent recruitment, and active confrontation of negative comments about psychiatry's image, to name but a few (Taintor and Robinowitz, 1981). The implementation of many of these recommendations has improved recruitment considerably, with 4.3 percent of United States medical school seniors matching into first-year positions in 1987. It is reasonable to expect that more than five percent of all United States students will enter the field (at the first and second postgraduate years combined) in the near future.

Other issues are likely to affect the composition and recruitment of those choosing psychiatry. Medicine in general appears to be evolving into a less attractive profession, as demonstrated by the fact there has been a drop in applications from 2.8 per position in 1973, to 1.9 in 1987 (Beeson, 1987). By 1990, it is estimated that there will be an applicant-position ratio of 1.5, the lowest in 60 years (Association of American Medical Colleges Weekly Report, 1987a). It is also important to note that the number of male applicants has declined steadily over the last 11 years by about 33 percent. During the last 15 years, however, women have been applying in increasing numbers: from 1500 in 1970, to 11,000 in 1984 (Swanson, 1986). Recent data from the NRMP indicates that some of the increase in applications to psychiatric training programs is related to the increasing numbers of women graduating from medical schools. Women appear to be significantly more likely to choose specialty training in obstetrics, pediatrics, pathology, or psychiatry than the other clinical specialties. Because there are so few data available, it is unclear whether this trend will be maintained in the long run or whether changes in the numbers of male applicants to psychiatry will occur. This is an area worthy of prospective study. The nation's 127 medical schools graduated 16,117 new physicians in 1986, 201 fewer than in 1985. Increasing tuition expenses and the substantial indebtedness by the time the doctor of medicine degree is acquired (averaging $34,000 per graduate, nearly $35,000 for those planning careers in psychiatry, 17 percent of the class of 1986 has debts in excess of $50,000) have been cited as important contributing factors (Association of American Medical Colleges Weekly Report, 1987a). Moreover, federal support of health manpower education is increasingly under attack (Iglehart, 1986). It is likely, however, that a more negative public image of medicine, increasing dissatisfaction of practitioners, increasing government regulatory intrusion in the practice of medicine, malpractice problems, and the oversupply of physicians also have an impact on this issue.

Manpower issues are complicated by decreasing support for undergraduate psychiatric education and the simultaneous increased need for faculty to generate income (Kay, 1987a). Directors of medical student education in psychiatry consistently identify insufficient numbers of teachers and generalized lack of teaching support and recognition as being critical and persistent problems (Cavanaugh and Kay, 1987). These concerns are especially relevant in light of many of the recommendations of the General Professional Education of the Physician (GPEP) Report (Mueller, 1984) for stronger efforts in psychosocial instruction and small group teaching.

Recruitment is likely to be influenced, although to what extent is unclear, by other factors, such as the physician surplus and the role of primary care practitioners in delivering mental health services. The field will also need to attend to the development of more systematic career pathways, beginning in medical school, to equip students with necessary basic neuroscience research skills that will enable them to be productive researchers within psychiatry. Significant financial support for M.D.-Ph.D. programs will be vital.

Many of the new forces acting on psychiatry have been briefly reviewed. These include significant changes in economics, training support, practice settings and patterns, need for psychiatric services, and general medical education. With these in mind, what will the future of psychiatric education entail?

The Future of Psychiatric Education

Selection

Any discussion of the future of undergraduate and graduate psychiatric education must logically begin with the selection process. New economic forces and the recent recruitment problems in psychiatry initiated an important examination by the American Psychiatric Association, the Residency Review Committee in psychiatry, the American Board of Psychiatry and Neurology (ABPN), and the American Association of Directors of Psychiatric Residency Training (AADPRT) of the quality of psychiatric training. The goal of this review was to improve the quality of resident applicants, assure increased quality of training programs, and decrease the variability in the quality of graduates (Kay, 1987b). In 1982, the American Psychiatric Association Task Force to Study the Quality of Residency Training in Psychiatry was created. It was charged with reviewing the overall patterns of training, the accreditation process of training programs, the quality and number of residents and their learning experiences, funding approaches, and recruitment procedures.

This task force reaffirmed important selection issues already under consideration by the Residency Review Committee and ABPN, most of which have been implemented through recent revisions in the Residency Review

Committee Essentials and ABPN requirements for certification. There was considerable concern that unqualified candidates, without adequate basic science and clinical education, were entering training, and that possession of a license to practice in a candidate's country of origin or passing the Educational Commission for Foreign Medical Graduates (ECFMG) did not necessarily provide such assurance. As a result, the new ABPN regulations and the Residency Review Committee Essentials require an Accreditation Council for Graduate Medical Education (ACGME)-approved first year of broad-based postgraduate training with specified primary care and neurology experiences. Similarly, the ABPN now requires all osteopathic physicians to successfully complete an ACGME-approved internship in addition to an osteopathic first postgraduate year, should the candidate wish to maintain doctor of osteopathic medicine certification eligibility. The new Essentials also require a trainee to have sufficient command of the "American language and culture," as well as having a sufficient command of English, to ensure accurate and unimpeded communication with patients and teachers. If residents are transferring from another program, their new program must be individualized so that all educational requirements have been met.

Under the new Essentials, residency training directors, assisted by residency selection committees, are specifically charged with establishing a process of recruiting only those who are personally and professionally suited for psychiatric training. They are also required to document selection procedures, including the checking of credentials, specific clinical training experiences, past performance, and professional integrity of trainees transferring from another program (including those entering at the child psychiatry fellowship level).

While as yet not incorporated into the Essentials, the American Psychiatric Association task force recommended that all programs require of their applicants the successful completion of a psychiatry clerkship conforming to the "Guideline for a Medical Student Curriculum in Psychiatry and Human Behavior" published by the American Psychiatric Association Committee on Medical Student Education (American Psychiatric Association, 1982). While such a clinical experience is a traditional component of United States medical schools, many foreign medical schools do not offer or require a clinical clerkship in psychiatry.

Foreign medical graduates are likely to enter all specialty training in this country in greatly reduced numbers. The entry requirements for the ECFMG have become more rigorous, and the Foreign Medical Graduates Examination in Medical Sciences (FMGEMS) exam has proven to be quite challenging. In the near future, it is anticipated that a clinical skills examination will be required of all seeking graduate training in this country. Moreover, there has been a major effort to examine the quality of Caribbean medical schools, which enroll a substantial number of American students unable to enter American schools. Some states already prohibit residency training for graduates of these schools; other states have moved toward refusing licensure to all foreign medical graduates.

Recent efforts by the AADPRT, with the support of many groups, have developed a selection process that will match all interested United States seniors into postgraduate year I or postgraduate year II positions in all of the country's psychiatry programs through the NRMP. This new process, to be effected in 1987 to 1988, will ensure ethical procedures for all medical student applicants, thereby removing considerable pressure and frustration in the selection process. This development is also consistent with the aims of the Committee on Graduate Medical Education and Transition from Medical School to Residency (Association of American Medical Colleges, 1987c), to lessen the disruptive effects of the selection process on the undergraduate medical education experience. The Association of American Medical Colleges has recommended improvement in the quality of dean's letters, appropriate use of National Board of Medical Examiners (NBME) test scores, the restraint on excessive audition electives, and a movement toward institutional responsibility in selection for all programs within a given institution.

While much has been accomplished recently to enhance the rigor of the selection process, many programs have not developed educational, characterological, and intellectual criteria for admission. Moreover, depending on the size of the applicant pool and institutional service needs, some programs may lower their criteria for admission. A strong future for psychiatric education will require increasingly sophisticated entry requirements. Considerable sentiment has developed recently for the return of a transitional year internship.

The New Residency Curriculum

The rise of corporate medicine and the creation of new practice settings, the surplus of physicians, the increasing government demand for accountability, the intense competition for the mental health care dollar, the growing needs of the chronically mentally ill in the public sector, and the explosive developments in neuroscience and its applied technology are creating significant tensions within the residency training curriculum. These tensions can be summarized by the following questions: 1) Will new models for instruction be required? 2) Should residents be prepared for new practice settings and how? 3) Should psychotherapy maintain centrality in the curriculum? 4) With expansion of knowledge, will psychiatry evolve into greater subspecialization, and if so, how should the resident prepare for this? 5) How should the quality of training programs and the trainees be monitored?

Toward a New Model

Given the certainty of a persistently expanding knowledge base and evolving practice settings, the new curriculum must preserve traditionally effective clinical and teaching experiences, while incorporating innovations that will foster life-long attitudes and skills for continuing education. Even amidst all of the changes in psychiatry, however, it is likely that clinical experiences, individual supervision of these experiences, and didactic seminars will remain at the core of resident education (Langsley, 1987; Taintor, 1987). There can be no substitute for well-conceived and well-supervised, phase-appropriate learning experiences with patients. The important educational task is determining how much of and which specific experiences should be required of the resident. The results of a 1986 survey show that individual institutions develop solutions depending on department philosophy, faculty resources, and service demands (Tasman and Kay, 1987). Excluding the internship year, only four clinical experiences are offered by nearly every program: adult inpatient work, outpatient rotations, child and adolescent psychiatry, and consultation–liaison psychiatry. Of these, only inpatient psychiatry is essentially a full-time rotation, as over 50 percent of programs offer child, outpatient, and consultation–liaison psychiatry as quarter or half-time rotations. Of equal importance was the fact no other rotation is offered by over 50 percent of the programs. Less than 25 percent of the programs responding required rotations in forensic, administrative, geriatric, or specialized inpatient psychiatry. Less than 10 percent of residencies required experiences in partial hospital settings. These data indicate that individual programs are already making decisions regarding which specific areas of subspecialty knowledge should be required. As the knowledge base increases, leading to further subspecialization among members of academic faculties, there will be increased pressure from both accrediting bodies and trainees to include a variety of areas of subspecialty training during the four-year residency program. It is already apparent that no program can offer subspecialty training in all areas, however defined, during residency training. This pressure may lead to new models of training that incorporate the need for a biphasic training program. One such model would consist of several years of training in a *core* curriculum, which every resident should experience, followed by elective opportunities in a variety of tracks, to provide the chance for residents to pursue areas of subspecialty interest prior to making decisions about fellowship training. At this time, there may not be a consensus regarding what constitutes a core curriculum and often decisions have been left exclusively to the Residency Review Committee's development of the Special Requirements for Training in Psychiatry. It seems likely that a more active and direct approach to determinations of core training activities will be required in the future. These are likely to take the form of critical-incident and time-and-motion studies.

Despite some concern over the viability of the academic health sciences center and the alleged attractiveness of new corporate-sponsored training sites, the most prudent course is to train for flexibility. It is unwise, however, to allow clinical training to be governed exclusively by delivery system changes, especially in a time when such changes are so rapidly evolving. Training for flexibility requires the introduction of new educational methodologies.

One fundamental method of promoting the capacity for future professional growth is via formal training in research. The aim of resident research experiences is to ensure that all psychiatrists possess the skills to evaluate research and incorporate research findings into clinical practice. A required and well-supervised experience in planning and/or conducting empirical research should include the following: critical literature review, hypothesis development, data acquisition plans (including comparative review of relevant instruments), data analysis plans, inferences, limitations, and conclusions (Nadelson and Robinowitz, 1987). While not all programs will be able to provide actual data collection experiences, the other components of a research curriculum should be easily implemented. Of course, training programs with substantial research resources should provide additional training to those residents, from both their own and other programs, who anticipate a professional research career.

As one of the pressures on today's training programs is to teach how to integrate new scientific knowledge, all residencies should require a level of computer literacy that permits the resident access to the scientific literature, databases, and other computerized information sources, such as bulletin boards. Such instruction will require programs to have computer and library resources and should become part of the accreditation requisites. Already the NBME has developed a computer-based exam, and it is likely that future licensing and specialty examinations will employ similar interactive video-disc formats, requiring the use of a microcomputer. Many hospitals employ microcomputers to record routine patient-management data (histories, physicals, laboratory test results) and the written medical chart may become obsolete. Computers can also enhance the learning of sound clinical management by enhancing the resident's ability to have at hand important data, for example, for tracking changes in medication doses across time. The increasing demand for faculty to generate portions of their salary may cause some programs to restrict their provision of individual supervision. While there must continue to be a minimal acceptable level, as mandated by the Residency Review Committee, this pressure may lead to a reexamination of other supervisory and learning models. Peer and group supervisory experiences have been underutilized for the most part in psychiatric training. This supervision format provides the additional advantage of a diversity of views, collegial support, and feedback mechanisms.

The use of self-study computer programs and interactive videotapes or videodiscs also holds promise for supporting some of the functions traditionally assumed by the didactic seminar. Interactive communications may be useful, ultimately, in teaching interview techniques as well. Furthermore, the importance of self-study techniques goes beyond the formal residency period. Computer assisted instruction should be one part of a departmental commitment to life-long educational efforts for both its residents and psychiatrists in the community.

In addition to providing innovative methods for training during psychiatric residency, these new technologies hold out tremendous potential for continuing education. As more and more health professionals have desk-top computers, either at home or in offices, the use of interactive teaching tools, based on either videotape or videodisc systems, seems likely to play an increasing role in the future of continuing education. It is possible that such technology will have an adverse impact on the popularity of attendance at Grand Rounds, lectures, or other traditional continuing education seminars.

Lastly, the federal government, through the National Institute of Mental Health, the National Institute on Drug Abuse, and the National Institute on Alcohol Abuse and Alcoholism, can be most helpful in assisting the assimilation of new scientific knowledge into the residency curriculum through 1) identifying new psychiatric research directions; 2) synthesizing research findings and their clinical relevance; 3) monitoring trends in clinical care, education, and research; and 4) supporting the development and dissemination of new training models. One area in which such assistance will be particularly important during training will be to provide residents with data synthesized from large-scale outcome and treatment efficacy studies. Pressures to contain costs will clearly have an impact on the clinical decision-making process, in that those treatment interventions shown to be correlated with positive outcome or a high likelihood of success must be learned and mastered by trainees. Psychiatry at present lags behind other specialties in the number of outcome studies available other than small-sample-size projects. It is clear that this state will not last for long and that these data must be incorporated into training in clinical decision making when it is available.

New Settings

The question of the role of new settings within the residency experience has been addressed in great detail in Chapter 2. Whether residents require actual training experiences in new settings is a major source of contention. Concerns have been raised about setting changes dictating new directions in clinical education, especially as they relate to ethical concerns within cost-containment conscious organizations such as health maintenance organizations. Others acknowledge that learning is facilitated when it takes place in clinical settings more predictive of where a trainee will eventually practice.

Ultimately, the soundest approach to this dilemma is one of requiring that all residents learn those skills essential to functioning in a multiplicity of settings. These skills need not necessarily be taught on site. As an example, skills required of a health maintenance organization's psychiatrist include supervising administration of psychotropic medication by primary care physicians; direct care of complex clinical presentations; facility with short-term treatment techniques; and supervision of mental health care givers. All of these skills can be, and have been, successfully taught in traditional settings.

Seminars (including readings and formal presentations from practitioners) on the varieties of practice should be a component of all training programs. The "Transition to Practice" seminar currently offered in most residencies should be broadened to include employment in newly developing settings. Of course, elective experiences should be developed in new settings with effective on-site and off-site supervision. Training directors must negotiate contracts in alternative settings that judiciously guard against residents being used for service needs exclusively. Resident programs are also encouraged to develop model affiliations between universities and new settings, where the goals are excellent patient care as well as new opportunities for research. One of the other impacts of an increased emphasis on economic efficiency in the health care system has been a decreased emphasis on primary and tertiary prevention. This clearly has an effect on residency training experiences, in that residents often focus most on alleviating the effects of an acute episode of illness, with a decreased emphasis on primary prevention or on alleviating the long-term after-effects of severe mental illness. It will be important, as economic pressures continue, to preserve such training experiences in primary prevention as providing residents the opportunities to evaluate offspring of parents hospitalized for psychiatric problems.

The Place of Psychotherapy

There have been many debates recently at national meetings regarding the centrality of psychotherapy in the future clinical practice of psychiatry. One reason for the intensity surrounding this issue is condensed in the fact that 70 percent of psychiatric practice time is currently devoted, at least in part, to psychotherapy (Langsley, 1987). Any reassessment, therefore, of the role of psychotherapy in the future practice of psychiatry may be, to a certain extent, anxiety provoking to current practitioners. Yet there is significant pressure on today's training program because of the need to integrate the rapidly expanding knowledge base in the neurosciences and clinical psychiatry. As the training experience could not be lengthened, psychotherapy instruction has been decreased in many programs. Indeed, according to a 1986 survey of 109 residency programs, more than 50 percent of them no longer offer long-term psychotherapy opportunities across the curriculum, but restrict psychotherapy experiences to circumscribed outpatient rotations (Tasman and Kay, 1987). Competition from other mental health disciplines has also led to questions regarding the uniqueness of psychiatry within the delivery of psychotherapy services. Additionally, the lack of long-term psychodynamic therapy outcome studies has raised cogent scientific questions about continuing to justify psychotherapy as *the* central skill in the residency program.

Through the examination of the psychotherapy issue, other fundamental pedagogical questions have surfaced: How should a resident be educated and trained for psychological understanding? Can this be done through activities other than psychotherapy? What skills beyond competent interviewing are required of tomorrow's psychiatrist within the doctor–patient relationship and as a consultant or administrator? Is there anything essential to the professionalization of the resident in having a long-term (approximately 24 months) intensive psychotherapeutic relationship with patients?

While economic forces, new settings, and increasing scientific knowledge will unquestionably alter some aspects of psychiatric practice, a depth psychological approach to the patient and his illness will always remain a key part of the fundamental clinical stance. Indeed, there are already concerns that the field has been so attracted to an exclusively biological approach to patient care that many of the significant insights of this century will be forgotten. Psychotherapy skills will be *one* of the core or essential skills for future psychiatrists, and long-term individual psychotherapy experiences should remain an important, although not as intensive, component in the training program. Despite the paucity of long-term psychotherapy efficacy studies, there are significant educational advantages for residents having these supervised experiences. They include: 1) an understanding of human development and the impact of early life experiences; 2) an appreciation of the process of psychic change and curative factors; 3) a preparation for understanding and handling intense affective states on the part of patient and therapist; 4) an illustration of the universality and clinical importance of distortions (transference) brought to the doctor–patient relationship by both parties; 5) an understanding of the nature of noncompliance and its applicability to all clinical work; and 6) the provision of an opportunity to observe closely the natural course of an illness.

In addition to long-term experiences, residents will need to master couple, family, and group treatment modalities. Greater attention will be devoted to conceptualized brief treatments (not those merely the result of forced termination due to rotational changes). These will be increasingly important not only because of economic reasons, but because of the growing scientific evidence of their effectiveness for specific disorders. In fact, there already appears to be evidence accumulating that family therapy has a positive impact on the outcome of treatment of patients with schizophrenia (McGill and Lee, 1986). Other studies seem to indicate the potential for similar effectiveness in patients with depression, eating disorders, and substance abuse.

Despite the decreasing attractiveness of psychoanalysis per se, most training programs will continue to emphasize a psychodynamic orientation in teaching therapeutic technique and theory. Of the 109 programs surveyed recently, 86 described their theoretical orientation for outpatient experiences as psychoanalytic, 20 as eclectic, and only one as cognitive (Tasman and Kay, 1987). However, tomorrow's psychiatrist will require facility in behavioral and cognitive therapies as well, and a national program to develop audio-visual tapes in all of the psychotherapies would greatly facilitate the teaching and learning of psychotherapeutic treatments. Moreover, it will be important to ensure that residents have ample supervised clinical experiences with patients of all ages and across all clinical disorders if they are to function effectively in newly emerging settings. Psychotherapeutic management of patients in a diversity of settings—inpatient, outpatient, emergency, and consultation–liaison—will therefore continue to be a prominent requirement in all programs.

With increasing time constraints on all programs, new methods and approaches will be required to maximize the quality and accuracy of supervisory methods. Studies should be undertaken to comparatively evaluate the traditional individual supervisory model drawn largely from psychoanalytic training and newer models of observation (live or by tape) of residents conducting psychotherapy. Greater attention will be focused on the evaluation of supervisor competence than has been the case in the past. Under persistent tensions about what to include in the curriculum, training programs will also devise new pedagogical methods to permit greater generalization of individual, group, and family psychotherapy experiences through requiring conceptually rigorous formulations beyond traditionally utilized case reports, discharge summaries, and dynamic formulations. Training programs will also move toward greater specification and evaluation of resident competence in the conduct of psychotherapies, for instance by requiring residents to supply audio-visual tapes of their treatments, and will systematically integrate new therapy procedures derived from psychotherapy research efforts.

During these times of rapid change within psychiatry, intensive reevaluation of traditional clinical and teaching models is taking place. This is an appropriate process, because time-consuming educational and clinical practices, such as those required in the conduct of psychotherapy, should not be endorsed without reasonable assessment. On the other hand, the current absence of efficacy data on certain psychotherapies should not lead to wholesale dismissal of the importance of psychotherapy skills in the future practice of psychiatry nor to the demise of psychotherapy instruction in the residency curriculum. While it is true that, in an atmosphere of increasing support of subspecialization, competency in psychotherapy may become a postresidency career course, but, for the forseeable future, the teaching and learning of psychotherapy will continue to be a highly important component in the residency training program.

Training for the Generalist and Subspecialist

Chapters 3 and 4 address perhaps the most debated issue in psychiatry today: Should the psychiatrist of the future be trained as a generalist or subspecialist? The argument for continuing to train generalists emphasizes that changing economic forces, shifting population needs, new settings, and an abundance of physician and nonphysician competitors require a clinical flexibility that can only be obtained through a broad-based education and training. Moreover, many argue that a de facto specialization has already taken place in some clinical areas and that formal subspecialization recognition is therefore unnecessary. There are concerns too that development of formal subspecialties within psychiatry would place generalists at a disadvantage, for example, in the eyes of the court, because they would not be seen as "experts." Similarly, many fear that generalists performing identical clinical work would create a higher risk of malpractice liability than formally recognized subspecialists. In terms of referral patterns, some also question whether large numbers of subspecialists could survive economically. In addition, subspecialization, in the minds of some, threatens the comprehensive or holistic approach to the clinical complexities of many psychiatric patients, with the possibility that other medical (family practice and internal medicine) and nonmedical (social work, psychology, family and marital counselors) practi-

tioners would assume the care of well-defined categories of patients traditionally under the care of psychiatry.

Arguments for the specialist approach consider chiefly the rapidly
expanding knowledge base of the field and the need to ensure that all trainees
have this new information and skills. Such teaching, it is proposed, can best
be taught by faculty with demonstrated expertise in special areas. As competition for psychotherapy patients and gatekeeping activities by primary care
physicians in health maintenance organization settings will threaten the position of psychiatry, a movement toward specialization would enhance the scientific base and visibility of psychiatry. At the Raleigh conference (April
3–4, 1986, Raleigh, North Carolina), a new model for educating the psychiatrist was proposed that contained both a core, or generalist phase of training,
and a specialist segment (Nadelson and Robinowitz, 1987). The former would
constitute the first three years of the residency, and the remaining year would
provide the resident with opportunities to concentrate in areas where special
knowledge and skills could be accrued. Requirements and qualifications for
offering such areas of concentration were described, as was the eventual
establishment of board certification for a given clinical area. It is argued that
such specialization opportunities would enhance the quality of psychiatric
training through teaching from acknowledged experts, provide graduates
with more marketable skills, and encourage referrals and consultation among
psychiatrists.

Quality of Training

As noted previously, the 1980s have been a period of intense review of
the quality of residency training programs by the Residency Review Committee, ABPN, the American Psychiatric Association, and AADPRT. This process has focused on selection criteria, accreditation, and trainee evaluation,
and it will continue to be a significant characteristic of training programs in
the future. The Residency Review Committee is the specialty component of
the ACGME responsible for developing and monitoring the Special Essentials
for Psychiatry, which describe the requirements with respect to form and content of psychiatry programs. This year, newly revised and more specific
Essentials, which highlighted many important concerns in the accreditation
process, were instituted. Increasing specificity with regard to length of rotations, practice settings, and types of patients treated, for example, drew some
objections that too-specific requirements might limit the creativity and the
local resources of a particular program. Residency Review Committee members, on the other hand, argued that, without highly circumscribed requirements, it is extremely difficult to disaccredit poor programs. The central
issue, then, is whether Residency Review Committee Essentials mandate
increasingly specific clinical experiences and learning activities, or establish
broad goals and standards permitting maximum program flexibility.

The implementation of the Essentials in any given training program is
evaluated through a regularly scheduled site visit, traditionally performed by

nonphysicians or by physicians, who may or may not be psychiatrists. The accreditation process in the future will rely more and more on psychiatrists for both routine site visits and those involving programs on probation. Moreover, it is likely that the next version of the Essentials will stipulate new faculty requirements with respect to specific faculty–trainee ratios and require evidence that faculty reflects a breadth and distribution of orientations, skills, and clinical and scientific interests. In addition, faculty will be formally assessed regarding their own professional growth, as represented by scholarship, research, clinical excellence, and public service. The quality of training will also be enhanced through the development of more specific knowledge, skills, and clinical experience requirements, as well as more rigorous examination and documentation of trainee progress and advancement. Training programs will increasingly utilize individual course examinations, in-service faculty-observed clinical examinations, and basic competency examinations. Successful completion of this last evaluation mechanism would become a prerequisite for graduation. In addition, a nationally sponsored cognitive exam, such as the Psychiatric Residents In-Training Examination (PRITE), is likely to continue to provide a vehicle for evaluating residents within and across training programs, while also permitting evaluative comparisons of programs with each other.

Undergraduate Psychiatric Education

New Forces in Medical Student Education

It is not surprising that the economic and knowledge issues impinging on graduate education are also becoming influential in medical student education. The long-awaited GPEP report, "Physicians for the Twentieth Century" (Mueller, 1984), produced recommendations for the general professional edu cation of tomorrow's medical student. It was the culmination of two years of testimony from 83 medical schools, 32 colleges and universities, and 21 medical professorial societies. The GPEP panel concluded that fundamentally little has changed in the way medical students are educated since Flexner's time. Strong criticism was expressed regarding the current information-intensive lecture format of nearly all medical schools. The GPEP panel advocated a greater emphasis on self-directed, independent learning, to prepare future practitioners for the rapidly increasing explosion in biomedical information and technology, as well as for the revolutionary changes in the manner in which medical care is to be delivered. While the recommendations of this report were considered to be sound, little change has been evident since its publication.

In addition to the GPEP's criticism of premedical and preclinical education, increasing concern has been voiced about the clinical education of students, especially with respect to ensuring that all acquire proficiency in the fundamental skills of clinical practice (Report of the National Invitational Conference, 1986). A number of forces are affecting the quality of clinical experiences for junior and senior students: 1) shortened length of hospital stay; 2) complexity of medical problems of those patients in teaching hospitals; 3) increasing reliance on technology for both diagnosis and treatment; and 4) reduction in availability to students of teachers because of increasing pressures to provide direct patient care to generate faculty salaries. The impact of cost-containment practices, such as diagnosis related groups, has faculty concerned that medical students are not provided the time to get to know their patients as people, study their medical presentations, appreciate the importance and intricacies of the doctor–patient relationship, or observe the natural course of illnesses, all of which can seriously interfere with the student's ability to accrue the values and attitudes that make physicians healers rather than data collectors and manipulators of technique (Association of American Medical Colleges, 1986b). Because of an emphasis on teaching from a biopsychosocial perspective, departments of psychiatry are in a unique position to provide input into clinical training in other sites and other specialties. Many of the concerns expressed regarding deficits in the training of students to be "healers rather than technicians" can be provided by a variety of programs integrated into the clinical training in settings other than psychiatric services. Of course, such teaching requires financial support and is often one of the first components of undergraduate curriculum to be cut when resources become limited. Ambulatory teaching sites will become more and more prominent in the clinical biennium, although funding such experiences are enormously costly. It has been estimated that it requires $15,000 per student year to offset the revenue loss from education in ambulatory clinics (Association of American Medical Colleges, 1986a).

Another significant challenge to undergraduate medical education is the introduction of medical information management. The rapidly evolving knowledge base of medicine will require that future physicians be able to store, retrieve, correlate, interpret, and manage clinical information. Today's reliance on textbooks, journals, patient charts, and the physician's memory to inform the clinical decision-making process will give way to greater reliance on *medical informatics*, or medical information science. The major obstacles to moving the curriculum in this direction are two: funding for development and on-site implementation of such programs and changing time-honored faculty values and attitudes about instructional methods.

All of the recommendations for revising the undergraduate curriculum will require an investment in energy and money more recently absent from this aspect of medical education. The reconceptualization, implementation, and administration of a vital and cohesive medical student education will require a significant modification of the traditional departmental-fiefdom model with which most medical schools currently struggle.

Medical Student Education in Psychiatry

At a time when there is significant and positive reevaluation of the importance of psychosocial instruction in the education of medical students

(Mueller, 1984), psychiatry departments are struggling with decreasing financial resources for medical student teaching (Kay, 1987b). Moreover, medical student educational activities continue to receive relatively low priority in many departments, despite the lessons taught via the recruitment problems of this decade. Medical student directors in psychiatry describe their most pressing problems as "1) not enough teachers or teaching time; 2) over-committed, overworked, burned out, and poorly motivated faculty; 3) lack of support, recognition, tenure, and monetary rewards for committed teachers; and 4) insufficient funding for psychiatric undergraduate medical education" (Cavanaugh and Kay, 1987). Amidst the intense concern over the funding and quality of graduate education, it will require a hypervigilance on the part of departmental chairs, colleges of medicine, and national psychiatric organizations to preserve the gains made over the last seven years in psychiatric medical student education.

In addition to the general forces impinging on all of undergraduate medical education, undergraduate psychiatric educators will be responding to the important changes in psychiatry as a field and those occurring within the psychiatric residency training program. What would be the potential impact on undergraduate psychiatry instruction and resident recruitment, for example, should other specialties like family medicine begin to offer programs certifying special competence in behavioral or psychological medicine? New activities and educational efforts, such as the development of special seminars in the integration of neurobiology and psychology, will be required to promote neuroscience interests in medical students, so that they will choose to become qualified researchers within the field.

The move toward subspecialization within psychiatric training programs is likely to alter undergraduate experiences in clinical psychiatry. Indeed, there are already tensions in the preclinical curriculum about what to include in behavioral science and psychopathology courses. Given the stricter limitations on lecture time in the preclinical curriculum, should psychiatric faculty utilize or emphasize their expertise in interviewing or should the focus be more on neurobiological advancements and their correlation to clinical understanding. Similarly, in the junior and senior clerkships, it is fairly common now for students to be assigned to specialty inpatient units (geropsychiatry, substance abuse, and so on,) for their only clinical encounter with psychiatry. Their assignment is determined not by considerations central to student education, but rather because residents are now being trained to ensure adequate exposure to important specialty areas. With more limited clinical exposure to general psychiatry, medical student educators must take thoughtful steps to ensure that students will receive a broad range of experiences suitable for the education of the primary care physician, as well as for sustaining those with career interests in psychiatry. With increasingly shorter patient stays in the hospital, it will be crucial that students not be overly preoccupied with diagnosis and disposition exclusively. They will need greater encouragement and supervision in appreciating the person behind the illness and universally helpful aspects of the doctor–patient relationship. With increasing clinical and administrative workloads for residents, there may be a tendency to inappropriately assign greater responsibility to students to meet service demands.

Psychiatry should consider innovative teaching methodologies for educating students about interviewing skills, psychopathology, psychopharmacology, and clinical decision making. Leadership in the development of interactive teaching devices is sorely needed. With a decreasing emphasis throughout all of medicine on inpatient work, the development of creative ambulatory rotations in psychiatry will be required. New clerkship sites should be explored as well. For example, training medical students in a health maintenance organization setting has been correlated with increased perceived quality of care and patient satisfaction, enhanced provider education, and greater provider practice satisfaction (Kirz and Larsen, 1986). However, the medical student teaching costs in health maintenance organizations may be considerable: 1) a decrease in productivity of 1.1 patient visits per half day; 2) direct physician teaching labor of 46.8 minutes per half day; and 3) an approximate cost of $16,900 per full-time equivalent student per year (Kirz and Larsen, 1986).

Departments of psychiatry, if they are to convey the richness and excitement of the field, should ensure that all students understand the functional neurobiology of the central nervous system and its effects on emotions and behavior; the role of psychological factors in all illness; basic psychopharmacology; human development; major psychopathological states and their appropriate treatments; and the importance of social, cultural, and environmental influences on the etiology, course, and treatment of illness. Students must be exposed to a wide range of theoretical and therapeutic models and should be required to master the basic diagnostic skills utilized in psychiatry. These include: 1) interviewing and history taking; 2) examining the mental status; 3) recognizing the major categories of mental illness and emotional disturbance; 4) organizing observable clinical data into a comprehensive formulation; 5) recognizing psychiatric emergencies; 6) appreciating the range of treatments offered by psychiatry; 7) recognizing the appropriateness and indications for referral to a psychiatrist; and 8) appreciating the psychiatrist as a consultant to other physicians (American Psychiatric Association, 1982).

Conclusion

Extraordinary forces are currently changing medical education and the practice of medicine. Psychiatry, like all other specialties, will be challenged by cost containment, the rise of corporate medicine, the surplus of physicians, and competition from other care providers. All of these issues are transforming the academic health science center and affiliated training sites into highly cost-conscious institutions that must create new funding mechanisms, teaching methods, and professional rewards if the practice of medicine, and psychiatry in particular, is to continue to be intellectually challenging. The future of psychiatric education will be one of integrating the exciting scientific advancements within new care settings, and ensuring that students and residents are adequately prepared to employ their clinical skills, regardless of where they practice.

References

Alper PR: Medical practice in the competitive market. N Engl J Med 1987; 316:337–339

American Psychiatric Association: A Guideline for a Medical Student Curriculum in Psychiatry and Human Behavior. Washington, DC, American Psychiatric Association, 1982

Asch DA, Parker, RM: The Libby Zion Case: one step forward or two steps backward. N Engl J Med 1988; 318:771–775

Association of American Medical Colleges: Council of Teaching Hospitals Survey of Housestaff Stipends, Benefits and Funding. Washington, DC, Association of American Medical Colleges, 1985

Association of American Medical Colleges: Medical Education: Institutions, Characteristics and Programs (background paper). Washington, DC, American Association of Medical Colleges, 1986a

Association of American Medical Colleges: Council of Teaching Hospitals Report, Vol 20, No 7, November 1986b

Association of American Medical Colleges Weekly Report, Vol 1, No 4, December 18, 1986c

Association of American Medical Colleges Weekly Report, Vol 1, No 13, February 26, 1987a

Association of American Medical Colleges Weekly Report, Vol 1, No 13, March 5, 1987b

Association of American Medical Colleges: Improving the Selections of Residents: An Agenda for Action. Washington, DC, Association of American Medical Colleges, 1987c

Beeson PB: Making medicine a more attractive profession. J Med Educ 1987; 62:116–125

Berrien R: What future for primary care private practice? N Engl J Med 1987; 316:334–337

Cavanaugh SA, Kay J: Problems in Undergraduate Medical Education in Psychiatry. Journal of Psychiatric Education 1987; 11:157–170

The Commonwealth Fund: Report of the Task Force on Academic Health Centers: Prescription for Change. New York, The Commonwealth Fund, 1985, pp III, 16

Ginsberg E: The monetarization of medical care. N Engl J Med 1984; 310:1162–1165

Goldman HH, Adams NH, Taube CA: Deinstitutionalization: the data demythologized. Hosp Community Psychiatry 1983; 34:129–134

Goldman HH, Ridgely S: The future environment for psychiatry, in Future Directions for Psychiatry. Edited by Talbott JA. Washington, DC, American Psychiatric Press, Inc., 1989

Guggenheim FG, Nadelson CN: Earn-as-you-go pressures in academic psychiatry. Am J Psychiatry 1984; 141:1571–1573

Iglehart JK: Federal support of health manpower education. N Engl J Med 1986; 314:324–329

Kay J: Economic issues and the undergraduate curriculum, in Training Psychiatrists for the 90's: Issues and Recommendations. Edited by Nadelson CC, Robinowitz CB. Washington, DC, American Psychiatric Press, Inc., 1987a, pp 191–198

Kay J: Selection processes for psychiatric residency, in Training Psychiatrists for the 90's: Issues and Recommendations. Edited by Nadelson CC, Robinowitz CB. Washington, DC, American Psychiatric Press, Inc., 1987b, pp 41–42

Kirz HL, Larsen C: Costs and benefits of medical student training to a health maintenance organization. JAMA 1986; 256:734–739

Kralewski JE, Dowd B, Feldman R, et al: The physician rebellion. N Engl J Med 1987; 316:339–342

Langsley DG: The education of tomorrow's psychiatrists, in Training Psychiatrists for the 90's: Issues and Recommendations. Edited by Nadelson CC, Robinowitz CB. Washington, DC, American Psychiatric Press, Inc., 1987, pp 63–70

McGill CW, Lee E: Family psychoeducational intervention in the treatment of schizophrenia. Bull Menninger Clin 1986; 50:269–286

More Companies Manage Mental Health Care Costs. Psychiatric News, March 4, 1988, p 18

Mueller S: Physicians for the twenty-first century, report of the project panel on the general professional education of the physician and college preparation for medicine. J Med Educ 1984; Vol 59, Part II

Nadelson CC, Robinowitz CB: Training psychiatrists for the '90s, in Training Psychiatrists for the 90's: Issues and Recommendations. Edited by Nadelson CC, Robinowitz CB. Washington, DC, American Psychiatric Press, Inc., 1987, pp 3–6

Petersdorf RG: A proposal for financing graduate medical education. N Engl J Med 1985; 312:1322–1324

Regier DA, Goldberg I, Taube CA: The defacto mental health service system. Arch Gen Psychiatry 1978; 35:685–693

Relman AS: Who will pay for medical education in our teaching hospitals? Science 1984; 226:20–23

Relman AS: The changing climate of medical practice. N Engl J Med 1987; 316:333–334

Report of the National Invitational Conference on the Clinical Education of Medical Students. J Med Educ 1986; Vol 61, Part II

Rieselbach RE, Jackson TC: In support of a linkage between the funding of graduate medical education and care of the indigent. N Engl J Med 1986; 314:32–35

Rogers D, as quoted in Warren JV, Plumb DN, Trezbiatowski GL: A crisis in medical education: thoughts on listening to a conference on medical education for the 21st century. JAMA 1985; 253:2404

Schiff RL, Ansel DA, Schlosser JE, et al: Transfers to a public hospital: a prospective study of 467 patients. N Engl J Med 1986; 314:552–557

Schwartz WB, Newhouse JP, Williams AP: Is the teaching hospital an endangered species? N Engl J Med 1985; 313:157–162

Shortell SM, Hughes EF: The effects of regulation, competition, and ownership on mortality rates among hospital inpatients. N Engl J Med 1988; 318:1100–1107

Swanson AG: United States medical school applicants and matriculants, 1960–1985 and beyond, in From Physician Shortage to Patient Shortage. Edited by Ginsberg E. Boulder, CO, Westview Press, 1986, pp 11–34

Taintor Z: Future residency programs will be rich in content, in Training Psychiatrists for the 90's: Issues and Recommendations. Edited by Nadelson CC, Robinowitz CB. Washington, DC, American Psychiatric Press, Inc., 1987, pp 71–73

Taintor Z, Robinowitz CB: The Career Choice of Psychiatry: A National Conference of Recruitment into Psychiatry. Journal of Psychiatric Education 1981; 5:157–178

Tasman A, Kay J: Setting the stage: residency training in 1986, in Training Psychiatrists for the 90's: Issues and Recommendations. Edited by Nadelson CC, Robinowitz CB. Washington, DC, American Psychiatric Press, Inc., 1987, pp 49–54

United States Department of Health and Human Services: Study of the Financing of Graduate Medical Education. Washington, DC, Arthur Young & Company, 1986

Chapter 8

The Cutting Edge: A Blueprint for Curriculum Change and Future Research in Psychiatry

Gordon Strauss, M.D.
Gayle E. Strauss, Ed.D.
Joel Yager, M.D.

The process of synthesis and integration is an important part of keeping pace with the growth and change in the field of psychiatry, and this is especially relevant for psychiatry training programs. An eclectic approach to psychiatric education requires that a variety of educational tasks be pursued in a resident's training (Yager, 1977), so the issue of allocating curriculum time and resources to different areas of the field has become more difficult. There is and will continue to be pressure on the curriculum to make room for the increasing knowledge resulting from advances in neuroscience. At the recent American Psychiatric Association-sponsored conference on training in the 1990's (Nadelson and Robinowitz, 1987), an entire session was devoted to examining whether residents in psychiatry should be trained as psychotherapists. The question highlights the dilemma for many psychiatric educators: unless training is lengthened, we may soon reach the limits of simply adding more to our curriculum. We will have to decide which didactic or clinical experiences we can reduce, make elective, or do without.

This question of which goals an educational program should seek to attain is an old one. In 1949, Ralph Tyler addressed this issue in his classic treatise on curriculum: "if an educational program is to be planned and its efforts for continued improvement are to be made, it is very necessary to have some conception of the goals that are being aimed at. These educational objectives become the criteria by which materials are selected, content is outlined, instructional procedures are developed and tests and examinations are prepared." (Tyler, 1949, p. 3). Tyler suggested that those responsible for the educational purposes of a program might look to three major sources to guide them: 1) the needs of society, 2) the psychology of learning, and 3) suggestions from subject specialists. Attention to the needs of society means that psychiatry should examine the threat of nuclear war, the plight of the chroni-cally mentally ill and homeless, the problems of drug addiction and alcoholism, and the unequal distribution of poverty. Research in the discipline of educational psychology has demonstrated that limitations exist as to how much an individual can learn in a given amount of time, and there are often tradeoffs between emphasis on breadth or depth in planning learning experiences. One also must consider the organization of learning experiences. They should be organized to reinforce each other, so that there is continuity, sequence, and integration. Recent proposals calling for an additional year of specialization reflect the ever pressing dilemma of deciding what should be *core* and what should be *specialty* in the psychiatric curriculum.

While all three of Tyler's sources of objectives are vital and necessary and should be integrated with each other, this chapter deals only with the third: suggestions from subject specialists. As part of a project designed to identify the "cutting edges" in psychiatry, we asked a distinguished group of psychiatric researchers and subspecialists to identify the important developments during the decade from 1970 to 1980, as well as important research questions for the current decade. Their answers for the field of psychiatry as a whole have been reported elsewhere (Strauss et al., 1984). Their views with respect to their individual areas of specialization provide a blueprint for future psychiatric curriculum revision, while the questions they identified as answerable constitute a research agenda.

Methodology

We developed a list of 40 specialty areas within psychiatry derived from the Comprehensive Textbook of Psychiatry (Kaplan et al., 1980). Members of the faculty of the University of California, Los Angeles (UCLA), Department of Psychiatry and Biobehavioral Sciences, supplied us with the names of experts other than themselves in their own specialty areas; this yielded a list of approximately 1200 names. These first 1200 also were asked about persons in their specialties whom they considered especially productive or important, and in this way we obtained another 250 names. Experts were sent a one-page questionnaire for their specialty area and an identical questionnaire for psychiatry as a whole. A second mailing was sent out to all nonrespondents after four months. We received 461 replies (32%) from the 1429 experts surveyed. At least partial answers to the specialty questionnaires were received from 300 (65%) of the respondents.

Of the 300 experts who responded by answering one or more specialty questionnaires, 93 (31%) responded in the biological areas and 112 (37%) responded in the psychosocial areas reported here. (Only topics with 10 or more respondents are reported.) Thirteen psychosocial categories have been condensed to seven because of considerable overlap in the answers from several logically related specialty areas. The categories which have been combined include: 1) Psychoanalysis *plus* Dynamic Theories of Personality and Psychopathology *plus* Borderline States and Personality Disorders; 2) Consultation–Liaison and Behavioral Medicine *plus* Psychophysiological Disorders and Chronopsychophysiology; 3) Community Psychiatry *plus* Social Psychiatry; 4) Psychotherapy *plus* Neurosis and Anxiety States; 5) Behavior Therapy *plus* the Application of Learning Theory and Biofeedback. These combined categories and two others, Normal and Abnormal Sexuality and The Family and Family Therapy, represent the categories in psychosocial psychiatry in which at least 10 experts responded.

We have organized the information by dividing the specialists' categories into biological and psychosocial topics. We realize these distinctions cannot be clear-cut in every instance. (The topics dealt with in this chapter omit obviously important areas, such as affective disorders. For this and other topics not included, we simply had too few specialists responding.) The individual subspecialists who participated in the survey are listed at the end of this chapter.

Biological Categories

Neurobiology and Behavior

Developments related to neuropeptides led the list of accomplishments in this category by a wide margin. Included were the discovery and characterization of endorphins and enkephalins, as well as the demonstration that certain peptides are common to the brain, gastrointestinal tract, and pituitary. Also included here were work on neuropeptides as transmitters and related studies of receptors. Another key area was the development of new techniques to map brain anatomy and metabolism, including the application of immunohistochemistry to the nervous system, and methods using 2-deoxyglucose and horseradish peroxidase. More clinical developments included noninvasive brain-scanning techniques, such as positron emission tomography (PET) or computerized tomography (CT); progress in the study of schizophrenia, including studies of dopamine and dopamine blockers; and clinical applications of basic research, such as urinary levels of 3-methoxy-4-hydroxyphenylglycol (MHPG) in mania, use of radioimmunoassay methods in psychotropic drug treatment and measurement of antidepressant plasma levels. Important developments in neuroanatomy included the discovery of pioneer fibers in invertebrates, the sensitivity of the visual cortex to environmental experience, and changes in the growth of corticodendrites with age. The isolation, synthesis, and study of the behavioral effects of hypothalamic hormones, as well as brain laterality research in animals and humans, were also highlighted.

For the future, the respondents in this category look for answers to some of the following questions about endorphins and other peptides: What is the mechanism of action of the peptides in the nervous system and elsewhere? How do "gut" or peripherally injected peptides affect the brain? Are enkephalins involved in psychosis? Is there a role for peptides in the treatment of schizophrenia or depression? How do opioid and nonopioid peptides interact? The neurobiologists also hope for greater understanding of relationships between brain and mind: What parts of the brain "work" during different mental states? What are the anatomical, physiological, and chemical bases of specific cognitive processes, such as learning and memory? Clinically, questions such as the following may be answerable: What are the genetic and biochemical bases of disorders such as schizophrenia, bipolar illness, and senile dementia? Predicted developments in psychopharmacology include safer, more rapidly acting antidepressants, techniques for more easily monitoring blood levels, a better understanding of the genetic influences on drug efficacy, and more effective behavioral/pharmacologic methods of patient management.

At a more basic level were questions such as: What is the molecular basis of cell recognition and of the specificity of neural connections? How does this develop embryologically? How many modes of cell interaction are there? What is the molecular basis of regeneration in the central and the peripheral nervous systems? What is the role of the cerebral cortex in the control of the immune system and how does it relate to genetic regulation of the body's immune response? How does brain biochemistry relate to central nervous system electrophysiology?

Basic and Clinical Psychopharmacology

A moderate amount of overlap with responses for the previous category was noted, not unexpectedly. Respondents in this category gave most emphasis to studies of neurotransmitters and receptors, including the development of technology to label and measure brain receptors, studies of histamine and H2 receptor blockers, studies of gamma aminobutyric acid (GABA), and the realization that peptides are brain neurotransmitters. The discovery of endorphins and endogenous opiate receptors was of course a major point. Developments in clinical psychopharmacology included the use of lithium in the treatment and prophylaxis of bipolar disorders and in schizoaffective illness, and improved understanding of drug actions such as the discovery of antidepressant effects of precursors of serotonin. Methodological advances in neurochemistry were given prominence, including studies of protein phosphorylation in the regulation of neuronal function, identification and behavioral studies of hypophysiotropic hormones, and the development of the deoxyglucose method to map brain metabolism. Clinically focused achievements included the development of biological markers, such as the dexamethasone suppression test, measurement of MHPG and prolactin, research on the uses of antidepressants for conditions such as panic disorder, the clinical use of serum measurements of medications, and demonstration of the value of long-term neuroleptic use in schizophrenia.

Like the neurobiologists, the pharmacologists expect many of the answerable questions to be in the areas of neuropeptides and neurotransmitters. They expect answers to such questions as: Can synthetic neuropeptides be used clinically as medications? What are the roles of neuropeptides, trans-

Table 1. Most Prominent Developments in Neurobiology, Psychopharmacology, and Schizophrenia

Developments in Neurobiology

Discovery of endorphins/enkephalins
Neuropeptides as transmitters
New techniques to study brain anatomy, metabolism
Studies of schizophrenia and dopamine
Better understanding of drug actions

Developments in Basic and Clinical Psychopharmacology

Studies of neurotransmitters and receptors
Discovery of endorphins/enkephalins
Uses of lithium

Developments in Schizophrenia

Advances in neurosciences
Advances in psychopharmacology
Advances in diagnosis
Studies of family environment and relapse

mitters, and receptor systems in the pathogenesis of schizophrenia and other psychiatric disorders? What is the function of neuropeptides and neurotransmitters in learning and memory and in disorders of these functions? There are two broad questions about diagnosis: Can diagnostic subclassification yield disorders with more specific treatments? Can biochemical markers be found to diagnose and monitor disorders such as depression and anxiety? The pharmacologists also hope to learn when it is valuable to measure blood levels of psychotropic drugs or their metabolites, and whether there is any clinical value in measuring neuroleptic blood levels. They also hope for a better understanding of the interaction of psychotherapy with pharmacotherapy, especially in the maintenance treatment of depression and personality disorders. Three questions complete this list: What are the mechanisms of action of lithium and antidepressants? Can a true antianxiety drug be developed that is not pharmacologically a sedative? By what mechanism does phencyclidine hydrochloride (PCP) cause altered mental states?

Schizophrenia

The experts in schizophrenia felt that the list of accomplishments for the past decade was led by developments in neuroscience. These included explorations of the dopamine theory and its limitations, discovery of endorphins and their receptors, basic research on the mechanisms of medication action at the cell membrane, and catecholamine research. Next most frequently mentioned were advances in psychopharmacology, including recognition of the risk of tardive dyskinesia from prolonged neuroleptic drug treatment, demonstration of the effect of maintenance neuroleptics on relapse rates, the possible role of propranolol as an antipsychotic, the identification of phenothiazine nonresponders, and the utility of lithium as an ancillary drug in schizophrenia. Advances in diagnosis and phenomenology included the International Pilot Study of Schizophrenia and the development of reliable, specific, and operational criteria for diagnosis; the shift toward a narrower concept of schizophrenia; and the working out of the natural history of schizophrenia, including the designation of characteristics associated with good and poor treatment response.

The influence of the family environment (for example, expressed emotion) on relapse was considered important, as was genetic research, including the role of adoption studies, in establishing and confirming a genetic basis for schizophrenia. Attempts to deal with chronicity, such as techniques of supportive care that include token economies and social learning approaches to rehabilitation, were also considered important. Studies of the brains of schizophrenics were given less emphasis; included here were CT evidence of structural changes in schizophrenia, the neurochemical investigation of postmortem brains, and the invention of PET scanning.

For the future, the specialists appear to be equally interested in questions about the biology and psychosocial aspects of schizophrenia. The biological questions include: Are there chemical or other biological markers for diagnosis or prognosis? Is there anything special about the pre- or postsynaptic receptors or their neurotransmittors in schizophrenia? Can studies be designed to combine adoption strategies with measures of family environment, so that we can say what kinds of families will produce schizophrenic offspring? Questions about psychological intervention and rehabilitation include: What is the best way to combine psychological management with medication? What special features are required for an inpatient milieu to facilitate the psychotherapeutic treatment of schizophrenic patients? Can we be systematic about selecting the most effective rehabilitation procedures for individual patients in remission? Other questions include: Can meaningful subtypes be identified, using biological markers or medication responsiveness? Can we predict which patients are at greatest risk for the development of tardive dyskinesia, as well as which patients can be maintained without medication? Under what conditions can family therapy or social skills training reduce relapse and/or contribute to improve prognosis? Are the structural changes in the brain that can be measured with CT scans a consequence of the disease?

Drug Dependence and Alcoholism

The specialists in this area were unanimous in naming the studies of endorphins and enkephalins and the discovery of the opiate receptor as the leading developments of the decade (Table 2). Two other developments were given prominence: studies of the effects of alcoholism in pregnancy, including research on the fetal alcohol syndrome, and the development of narcotic antagonists for clinical use. Developments in analytical clinical toxicology were highlighted, as was progress in the treatment of dependency and withdrawal.

In the decade of the 1980s, those working in the area of drug abuse and alcoholism hope to learn the physiological, cellular, and molecular bases of tolerance and physical dependence. Other questions of importance include: What is the role of endorphins in drug dependence? What are the mechanisms that predispose some people to develop alcoholism and what mechanisms protect other people from the same disease? Can we develop a satisfactory chemotherapy for alcoholism using alcohol antagonists or modulators? What is the role of narcotic antagonists in the treatment of opiate addictions? What are the most cost-effective treatment methods for drug and alcohol problems? Do alcoholics and nonalcoholics differ premorbidly in metabolic pathways or rate and manner of metabolism?

Electroconvulsive Therapy (ECT)

The development and study of unilateral and other electrode placements and studies of side effects, especially to memory, were mentioned most often by respondents in this area (Table 2). Improvements in equipment and studies of the relationship of current to seizure induction were considered important, as were neuroendocrine theories of the mechanism of action of ECT.

For the future, experts in ECT expect to learn more about the mechanism of effect in ECT, specifically about the relationship between physical parameters, such as wave form and current, and effectiveness or side effects.

Table 2.   Most Prominent Developments in Substance Abuse, Electroconvulsive Therapy, and Genetics

Developments in Drug Abuse and Alcoholism

Discovery of opiate receptor, endorphins/enkephalins
Studies of alcoholism in pregnancy
Narcotic antagonists for clinical use

Developments in ECT

Unilateral electrode placement
Systematic studies of effects on memory
Improved hardware
Neuroendocrine theories of how ECT works

Developments in Genetics

Adoption studies
New genetic models (and techniques to test them)
Laboratory methods to study and detect genes
Usefulness of genetics in clinical nosology

They hope to learn more definitively whether ECT produces long-lasting brain dysfunction and to what extent there are persistent memory deficits. Clinical questions of importance include: What are the predictors of therapeutic response to ECT? Under what conditions is ECT the treatment of first choice? Can ECT be replaced by more effective pharmacologic interventions? There are also questions about ECT's role in blood-brain barrier kinetics and in dopamine receptor subsensitivity.

Genetics in Psychiatry

Adoption studies and new genetic models and the techniques to test them (such as threshold models in the analysis of phenotypic heterogeneity) led the list of accomplishments in this category (Table 2). Laboratory methods for studying and detecting genes included amino acid sequencing, DNA insertion, and HLA grouping. The usefulness of genetics in clinical nosology was also highlighted and included the genetic classification of unipolar and bipolar affective disorders, as well as studies of genetic factors in schizophrenia and alcoholism.

The psychiatric geneticists expect the coming decade to lead to the discovery and identification of stable genetic markers of susceptibility to psychiatric disorders. They expect that, by using high-risk families, it will be possible to detect and analyze the interplay of environmental and cultural factors in psychiatric disorders. Other questions which may be answerable in the 1980s include: What is the genetic predisposition for drug abuse and alcoholism? Can homogeneous subforms of major syndromes be identified by conjugation and linkage analysis? Can refinements in the technique of studying adoptees be used to clarify the boundaries and essential characteristics of psychiatric disorders?

Psychosocial Categories

Psychoanalysis, Personality Disorders, and Dynamic Theories of Psychopathology

The work of Kohut conceptualizing disorders of the self and their treatment was the most frequently mentioned accomplishment of the past decade in this category (Table 3). This was followed by the work of Margaret Mahler, especially on separation and individuation, Kernberg's contributions on borderline and narcissistic disorders, and the contributions of child and infant observation research to our understanding of normal development and developmental arrests. Other accomplishments in relation to borderline conditions included Donald Klein's work in pharmacotherapy, Masterson and Rinsley's concept of pathogenesis, and adoption studies showing that relatives of schizophrenics have few characteristics in common with borderline patients.

In the future, the specialists in this area expect answers to the following questions: How do changes in technique growing out of the work of Kohut,

Table 3. Most Prominent Developments in Psychoanalysis and Personality, Consultation–Liaison, and Family Therapy

Developments in Psychoanalysis, Personality Disorders, and Theories of Psychopathology

Kohut's concept of self-disorders
Mahler's studies of separation and individuation
Kernberg's work on borderline and narcissistic disorders
Infant observation research

Developments in Consultation–Liaison and Behavioral Medicine

Use of behavioral techniques in clinical medicine
Growth of liaison psychiatry
Research on circadian rhythms
Acceptance of bio-psycho-social model for all illness

Developments in the Family and Family Therapy

Distinct approaches to family therapy
Increased coherence as a sub-specialty
Paradoxical techniques
Focus on the family system

Kernberg, and others affect the boundary between psychoanalysis and other forms of psychotherapy? How will self-psychology be integrated into psychoanalytic theory? Can psychoanalysis contribute to more sophisticated theories about affect and learning? What is the optimal treatment approach for personality disorders, including the role of medications in combination with psychotherapy? What are the dynamic and/or biologic relationships of personality disorders to other forms of psychopathology? Can a resolution be found to the controversy over *conflict versus deficiency* theories of pathogenesis? Can we observe new transference transfigurations that will advance both theory and technique for handling transference?

Other questions include: Can we refine our understanding of the emergence of early gender identity? What is the nature of the therapeutic process in psychotherapy? Can we develop appropriate research methods to study analytic processes and outcomes? What is the environmental contribution to borderline patients' difficulty in managing aggression? Can we identify the relative weights of stress (environment and diathesis), hereditary, and congenital determinants in the pathogenesis of personality disorders?

Consultation–Liaison and Behavioral Medicine

The application of behavioral methods to clinical medicine, including relaxation training and biofeedback, was the most frequently mentioned development in this category (Table 3). This was followed by the growth of liaison psychiatry, including National Institute of Mental Health support of training, increased support by community hospitals, and the spread of liaison nursing with the documentation of cost benefits. Efforts to understand circadian rhythms were highlighted, including the definition of two human circadian oscillators, the dependence of sleep architecture on the circadian phase of the temperature oscillator, studies of the role of the pineal in photoperiodism, the demonstration of neuroendocrine circadian rhythms, and the evidence that lithium slows circadian rhythms.

Among the other key accomplishments were developments in psychoimmunology, including the recognition of psychosocial influences on the immune system; studies of life stress, coping, and adaptation; professional and public interests in death and dying and the growth of the hospice movement; and psychological risk factors in cardiac disease, including studies of type A behavior.

There were several questions for the present decade about which there was considerable agreement. Experts in this area expect that the question of the effectiveness of consultation–liaison will be answered, and that part of this issue is whether consultation–liaison reduces the cost of medical care. Another key question for this decade is understanding the relationships between behavior, stress, and disease. In particular, the specialists expect the answers to the following two questions: What are the mechanisms by which stress contributes to disease? How does the immune system mediate between emotions and behavior and the development of cancer? The specialists also expect that the relationship of altered circadian rhythms to psychiatric illness in general and affective disorders in particular will be clarified.

Other questions in this area include: What are the limits of behavioral and social methods to effect changes in "lifestyles"? Can the public be educated to understand and accept psychophysiological self-regulation to ameliorate chronic health problems, with resultant decreased use of surgery and medications for these problems? Is is possible to develop a patient model that complements the disease model? Can we better understand depression in medical illness, so that more effective treatments can be developed? What are the genetic and environmental determinants of consumption disorders, such as alcoholism and obesity, and can subtypes be differentiated? Can rage, anxiety, and depression be differentiated on the basis of neuroendocrine patterns?

The Family and Family Therapy

Specific approaches to family treatment were the most frequently mentioned developments in this category; some of the approaches mentioned included Minuchin's structural approach, Haley's strategic therapy, brief family therapy, and developmental and intergenerational approaches (Table 3). Next most frequently mentioned was the growing coherence in the field of family therapy itself; included here were specific references to the development of the American Family Therapy Association, federal recognition of family therapy as an emerging discipline, the rapid growth in family therapy research publications, and the unification of the field as reflected in the Handbook of Family Therapy. The development of paradoxical techniques, notably by the Milan group, was mentioned often, as was the concept of systems and the chang ing focus from the patient to the family system.

For the coming decade, specialists in this area expect an improvement in the quality of research and look for the development of consensus about measures of process and outcome of family treatment. They hope for answers to such questions as: Can a family typology be developed and used for diagnosing family pathology? What in the theory and practice of family therapy really makes a difference? What is the most effective way to combine family therapy with other modalities, such as drug or individual therapy, or with other social supports? What are the relative contributions of genetics and family environment in the development of psychotic disorders? What is the impact of formal and informal supports, such as work or child care, on family functioning? How do constitutionally based individual differences interact with family characteristics or experiences in shaping development?

Other less frequently mentioned questions include: What is the impact of divorce and separation on child development? What are the factors that affect the incidence of child abuse? Do individual, long-term *talk* therapies really treat and ameliorate symptoms or merely stabilize family dysfunction?

Social and Community Psychiatry

The experts in this area emphasized developments in community psychiatric care, such as the continued evolution of mental health centers, catchmenting and the concept of continuous and comprehensive care, the development of long-acting neuroleptics, and the wide-spread use of nonphysicians to provide mental health services (Table 4). Aspects of deinstitutionalization and its backlash were important and included the recognition of the necessity of asylums, the issue of dangerousness, and the recognition of the value of hospital care within the spectrum of mental health treatments. The controversies about the roles of psychiatrists in community mental health centers and in the general care of chronic mental patients were included, as was the development of epidemiologic instruments to measure the frequency of affective disorders.

During the current decade, the specialists in community and social psychiatry expect that light will be shed on the nature of the ideal relationship between hospital and community care of chronic patients, with answers to such questions as: What will be the role of state hospitals in the mental health care delivery system? Is community treatment invariably the treatment of choice for chronic patients? Should hospitalization be equated with inadequate treatment of chronic patients? Can chronic patients be integrated into general hospital treatment settings? What aspects of community care represent advances over hospital care?

Another area where progress is expected is in studying the social determinants of chronic mental illness. Questions here include: Is schizophrenia less chronic in under-developed countries? Are the sex differences in the inci-

Table 4.   Most Prominent Developments in Social Psychiatry, Psychotherapy, Behavior Therapy, and Sexuality

Developments in Social and Community Psychiatry

Deinstitutionalization and its backlash
Developments in community care
Role of psychiatrist in CMH centers

Developments in Psychotherapy, Neurosis, and Anxiety States

Psychotherapy outcome research
Developments in brief psychotherapy
Exposure treatment for phobias and rituals
Manuals for cognitive and interpersonal therapies

Developments in Behavior Therapies

Cognitive behavior therapy
Clinical application of biofeedback
Defining the field's limits
Incorporation of systems theory

Developments in Normal and Abnormal Sexuality

Specific therapies for sexual disorders
Studies by Masters and Johnson
Objective measures of arousal

dence of depressive syndromes of primarily organic or social origin? What is the relation of environmental stress to the development of mental illness and is it true that social variables are only weak causes of the onset of most disorders? The experts are also concerned about the role of the psychiatrist in community mental health and whether effective professional relationships can be attained across mental health disciplines. Finally, the experts hope that the value and efficacy of prevention in psychiatry can be further clarified.

Psychotherapy, Neurosis, and Anxiety States

A majority of the specialists pointed to developments in psychotherapy research during the decade of the seventies (Table 4). These included the fact that few differences could be found when looking at outcome from different techniques with neurotic patients, clear evidence of the positive effects of therapy revealed in part by meta-analysis of psychotherapy studies, and objective instruments for measuring helping alliances. Developments in the technique and use of brief psychotherapy were considered quite important, as was the demonstration and acceptance of exposure treatments of phobias and compulsive rituals. Attempts to specify the content of certain forms of therapy, including the development of manuals for interpersonal and cognitive psychotherapy, were also highlighted.

For the current decade, experts in this area put emphasis on issues of outcome and process in psychotherapy. Questions about specific outcomes in psychotherapy include: Can outcome prediction be improved by looking at initial severity and/or process variables? What methods are most appropriate to study process and outcome? More specific process-oriented questions include: How should interventions be paced? How can patient and therapist be better matched? Which processes are most important in effecting change? Other questions that the experts in this area emphasized include: Can disorders and specific treatments be matched? What are the biological substrates of anxiety; for example, what neurotransmitters are primary and is there an endogenous *anxiogenic* substance? Can a model for combined psychotherapy and pharmacotherapy be developed? What is the relation of *neurosis* to organic illness and how can we use this relationship to learn more about the ways psychotherapy leads to decreased medical utilization? Will a better classification of *neurotic disorders* improve clinical practice? What is the role of short-term therapy, especially with borderline patients? Among the miscellaneous questions for the current decade are: When is conjoint marital treatment more or less effective than whole-family therapy? How do antidepressants and psychotherapy compare in the treatment of unipolar depression? Are there specific medications for panic states? What are the psychodynamic reasons for common state transitions? How should dynamic and cognitive/behavioral therapy be integrated?

Behavior Therapy

The emergence of cognitive behavior therapy (the manipulation of thought to change emotion and behavior) was the most frequently mentioned development of the decade from 1970 to 1980 (Table 4). This was followed by the clinical application of biofeedback, including its use in the treatment of anxiety, muscle-tension conditions, epilepsy, and stroke. Two other developments of importance were recognized: The incorporation of *systems theory* into behavior therapy with the application of behavioral techniques to nonclinical areas, such as energy conservation, and the use of exposure treatment (for example, flooding) for obsessive-compulsive disorders, anxiety, and grief.

The main question for the current decade is how valuable and effective can behavior therapies be with different disorders? Other more philosophical questions about behavioral work with patients include: What is the relationship of insight to action? What is the role of consciousness in behavior? To what extent is therapy an enterprise of morality and values? On a more practical level, how valid and viable is biofeedback and under what clinical circumstances? Several experts hope that there will be the development of a more adequate model for cognition, especially under conditions of stress. Among the miscellaneous questions for this decade are: Is the *instrument* necessary in behavioral medicine? How can social skills training be made more potent?

Normal and Abnormal Human Sexuality

Specific therapies for sexual disorders were mentioned most frequently by experts in this area (Table 4). The physiological observations and treatments of Masters and Johnson were mentioned often, as were the development and use of objective measures of arousal, such as nocturnal penile tumescence. Studies of normal development, including gender identity (and resultant revisions in psychoanalytic theory), were mentioned, as was the redefinition of homosexuality as nonpsychopathological. Also highlighted were confirmation that mammalian tissue is female until androgen is added, the elaboration of the dynamics of erotic excitement, and the identification of brain peptide-releasing factors and behavioral influences on hormones.

The experts in sexuality hope that the current decade will provide an understanding of the mental mechanisms of arousal, as well as new treatments for disorders of arousal. Their other questions include: What is the role of neurotransmitters in sexuality? How are sex and violence related? Can we develop theoretical models of sexual behavior that account for psychological, endocrinological, and neural variables?

Discussion

Our study focused on the cutting edge in both biologically and psychosocially oriented areas of psychiatry. What emerged first is a summary and reminder of the dramatic growth in biological psychiatry, as well as a research agenda for this decade (and probably much of the next as well). Clearly many underlying basic science discoveries have been important to these fields of psychiatry. The experts in neurobiology, psychopharmacology, schizophrenia, and substance abuse concurred in pointing to the developments and research in neuropeptides, transmitters, and receptors as the most important accomplishments within each of their fields.

For a decade or more the advances in neuroscience and in psychopharmacology have been the most well-publicized research developments in psychiatry (Freedman, 1980). This high visibility for biological research has had a number of salutary effects in balancing the public view of psychiatry, but psychiatric educators with a commitment to comprehensive training must also be aware of developments in the psychosocial areas of the field. As our data indicate, specialists in the psychosocial areas of psychiatry have as rich and varied a set of accomplishments and research questions as those in the biological areas. These data can be used to update basic curriculum and to help plan advanced and elective courses.

There are several educational implications from these findings for the instruction of medical students, psychiatric residents, and seasoned practitioners. While the revolution in biological psychiatry is given nearly universal lip service, and it is probably impossible to find a department of psychiatry which doesn't now teach psychopharmacology, more curriculum time devoted to basic and clinical neuroscience is warranted. Unless medical school psychiatry departments (and residency training programs) are willing to eliminate much of what they now teach, we may need to increase the total amount of curriculum time devoted to psychiatry and neuroscience. Training programs where the basic scientific foundation of current psychiatric knowledge is taught in depth are few and far between, though this is beginning to change.

At the same time that biological subject matter needs more curriculum time at both the medical school and residency levels of training, there are important new questions about what to teach within psychosocial psychiatry (Nadelson and Robinowitz, 1987). For example, how important is "self-psychology"? Is consultation–liaison psychiatry really worthwhile, or is it sufficient to teach residents a more purely consultation form of work in medical and surgical settings? Subspecialization in geriatrics and substance abuse appears likely, but will this trend extend to areas like family therapy? As forms of brief psychotherapy proliferate, how many are essential for general psychiatrists? For many of these questions there can be no single answer valid for all departments or all residency programs.

However, even more important for education and clinical practice in psychiatry is the convergence and overlap reflected in our results, at least in biological areas. At the same time as the knowledge base in biological psychiatry has become more detailed and subspecialized, there is increasingly a shared sense of what is important. It may be too soon to find an integration between biological and psychosocial areas in psychiatry, but we believe the outlines of an integrated biological psychiatry are starting to emerge. The rationale for an eclectic approach—the need for broadly based scholarship, for familiarity with current and unfolding information in diverse fields as a basis for the pragmatic use of a large repertoire of clinical skills—appears stronger than ever.

References

Freedman DX: Contempo 80: psychiatry. JAMA 1980; 243:2208–2210

Kaplan HI, Freedman AM, Sadock BJ (eds): Comprehensive Textbook of Psychiatry, 3rd edition. Baltimore, Williams & Wilkins Co., 1980

Nadelson CC, Robinowitz CB: Training Psychiatrists for the '90s: Issues and Recommendations. Washington DC, American Psychiatric Press, Inc, 1987

Strauss GD, Yager J, Strauss GE: The cutting edge in psychiatry. Am J Psychiatry 1984; 141:38–43

Tyler RW: Basic Principles of Curriculum and Instruction. Chicago, IL, University of Chicago Press, 1949

Yager J: Psychiatric eclecticism: a cognitive view. Am J Psychiatry 1977; 134:736–741

APPENDIX A

Respondents

Neurobiology

Bernard W. Agranoff, Ph.D.
Floyd Bloom, M.D.
W. M. Cowan, D.Phil.
David H. Coy, Ph.D.
Otto Creutzfield, M.D.
V. H. Denenberg, Ph.D.
David DeWeid, M.D.
Marian Diamond, Ph.D.
David Egger, Ph.D.
J. Engel, M.D., Ph.D.
Joaquin Fuster, M.D.
William F. Ganong, M.D.
Charles R. Hamilton, Ph.D.
Steven A. Hillyard, Ph.D.
Bartley Hoebel, Ph.D.
Turan M. Itil, M.D.
Karl H. Pribram, M.D.
Robert T. Rubin, M.D., Ph.D.
Andrew V. Schally, Ph.D.
Hans Selye, M.D.
E. A. Serafetinides, M.D.
Luigi Valzelli, M.D.
Herbert Weiner, M.D.
Roger S. Williams, M.D.
Robert J. Wyman, Ph.D.

Basic and Clinical Psychopharmacology

Ross J. Baldessarini, M.D.
Malcolm Bowers, Jr., M.D.
Magda Campbell, M.D.
Erminico Costa, M.D.
David DeWeid, M.D.
Edward F. Domino, M.D.
David L. Dunner, M.D.
David J. Greenblatt, M.D.
Frank D. E. Jones, M.D.
J. Korf, Ph.D.
Heinz E. Lehmann, M.D.
Herbert Meltzer, M.D.
Arthur Prange Jr., M.D.
Arthur Rifkin, M.D.
Robert C. Smith, M.D., Ph.D.
Fridolin Sulser, M.D.
Joseph Tupin, M.D.
Herman van Praag, M.D., Ph.D.
Theodore Van Putten, M.D.

Schizophrenia

Malcolm Bowers, Jr., M.D.
Timothy J. Crow, Ph.D., F.R.C.P.
Peter L. Giovacchini, M.D.
Solomon Goldberg, Ph.D.
Irving I. Gottesman, Ph.D.
James Grotstein, M.D.
John G. Gunderson, M.D.
John P. Leff, M.D., F.R.C. Psych.
Heinz E. Lehmann, M.D.
Robert P. Liberman, M.D.
Werner M. Mendel, M.D.
Thomas Ogden, M.D.
Gordon L. Paul, Ph.D.
Charles Schulz, M.D.
Helm Stierlin, M.D.
John Strauss, M.D.
E. Fuller Torrey, M.D.
Lyman C. Wynne, M.D., Ph.D.

Drug Abuse and Alcoholism

V. Charles Charuvastra, M.D.
Sidney Cohen, M.D.
Max Fink, M.D.
Alfred M. Freedman, M.D.
Ellen R. Gritz, Ph.D.
Y. Israel, M.D.
George D. Lundberg, M.D.
Peter E. Nathan, Ph.D.
Forrest S. Tennant, Jr., M.D.
Edward C. Tocus, Ph.D.
Carlton E. Turner, Ph.D.
Thomas Ungerleider, M.D.

ECT

T. George Bidder, M.D.
Giacomo d'Elia, M.D.
Max Fink, M.D.
Michel R. Mandel, M.D.
Carl Salzman, M.D.
Iver F. Small, M.D.
Lawrence Squire, Ph.D.
Michael Taylor, M.D.
George J. Wayne, M.D., Ph.D.
Lelon Weaver, Ph.D.
Richard Weiner, M.D., Ph.D.

Genetics

C. Robert Cloninger, M.D.
J. C. DeFries, Ph.D.
Lee Ehrman, Ph.D.
John Fuller, Ph.D.
Irving I. Gottesman, Ph.D.
J. Mendlewicz, M.D., Ph.D.
Theodore Reich, M.D.
David Rosenthal, Ph.D.
Paul H. Wender, M.D.

Psychoanalysis, Borderline States, and Personality Disorders

Dynamic Theories of Personality

Professor Herman Argelander
Samuel Eisenstein, M.D.
Rudolf Ekstein, Ph.D.
Willard Gaylin, M.D.
Arnold Goldberg, M.D.
James Grotstein, M.D.
John G. Gunderson, M.D.
Robert Langs, M.D.
Margaret Mahler, M.D.
J. F. Masterson, M.D.
Donald Meltzer, M.D.
David R. Metcalf, M.D.
Glen Miller, M.D.
George H. Pollack, M.D.
Leo Rangell, M.D.
Donald B. Rinsley, M.D.
Edward R. Shapiro, M.D
Robert J. Stoller, M.D.
Robert D. Stolorow, Ph.D.
Professor H. Strotzker
Marian Tolpin, M.D.
Robert S. Wallerstein, M.D.
Paul H. Wender, M.D.
Arlene Wolberg, M.D.
Ernest S. Wolpe M.D.

Consultation–Liaison Psychiatry and Behavioral Medicine

David Agle, M.D.
Paula Clayton, M.D.
Bernard H. Fox, Ph.D.
Elmer Green, Ph.D.
James P. Henry, M.D., Ph.D.
Jimmie Holland, M.D.
Jeffrey L. Houpt, M.D.
David Krantz, Ph.D.
Daniel F. Kripke, M.D.

Hoyle Leigh, M.D.
Z. J. Lipowski, M.D.
F. Patrick McKegney, M.D.
William C. Orr, Ph.D.
Gordon L. Paul, Ph.D.
Michael K. Popkin, M.D.
Daniel Schubert, M.D., Ph.D.
Edwin S. Shneidman, Ph.D.
Albert J. Stunkard, M.D.
John E. Upledger, D.O.
Anna Wirz-Justice, Ph.D.

The Family and Family Therapy

C. Beels, M.D.
Donald Bloch, Ph.D.
C. B. Broderick, Ph.D.
John Ewing, M.D.
Ira Glick, M.D.
Irene Goldenberg, Ed.D.
Michael J. Goldstein, Ph.D.
Edith H. Grotberg, Ph.D.
Reuben Hill, Ph.D.
Lynn Hoffman, A.C.S.W.
Bradford P. Keeney, Ph.D.
Michael Lamb, Ph.D.
Rudolph Moos, Ph.D.
Peggy Papp, A.C.S.W.
R. Ravich, M.D.
Robert G. Ryder, Ph.D.
Carlos E. Sluzki, M.D.
Ross V. Speck, M.D.
Peter Steinglass, M.D.

Social and Community Psychiatry

Ransom J. Arthur, M.D.
Roderic Gorney, M.D., Ph.D.
Milton Greenblatt, M.D.
Dr. A.S. Henderson
David Kinzie, M.D.
J. P. Leff, M.D., F.R.C.Psych.
Isaac Marks, M.D.
H. B. M. Murphy, M.D.
Donald Schwartz, M.D.
John Talbott, M.D.

Neurosis and Anxiety States, Psychotherapy

D. Wilfred Abse, M.D.
A. Bergin, Ph.D.
Sol L. Garfield, Ph.D.
Alan S. Gurman, Ph.D.

Mardi Horowitz, M.D.
E. Gartly Jaco, Ph.D.
Toksoz Byram Karasu, M.D.
Malcolm H. Lader, M.D.
Lester Luborsky, Ph.D.
David H. Malan, M.D., F.R.C.Psych.
P. E. Sifneos, M.D.
Marian Tolpin, M.D.
P. J. Tyrer, M.D., F.R.C.Psych.
Robert S. Wallerstein, M.D.

Behavior Therapy

T. D. Borkovec, Ph.D.
Gerald C. Davison, Ph.D.
Cyril Franks, Ph.D.
K. Gunnar Gotestam, M.D.

Leonard Krasner, Ph.D.
Isaac Marks, M.D.
Charles Wallace, Ph.D.
Joseph Wolpe, M.D.

Normal and Abnormal Human Sexuality

Paul R. Abramson, Ph.D.
Jack S. Annon, Ph.D.
Lonnie Barbach, Ph.D.
Donn Byrne, Ph.D.
Paul H. Gebhard, Ph.D.
H. S. Kaplan, M.D., Ph.D.
W. Charles Lobitz, Ph.D.
Jon K. Meyer, M.D.
D. C. Renshaw, M.D.
Robert J. Stoller, M.D.

Chapter 9

Reflections on the Future

Zebulon Taintor, M.D.

The purpose of this chapter is to offer some views that arise from a model of the future applied to the foregoing material. The model has two basic premises: 1) history can be divided into linear and cyclical phenomena; and 2) economic forces driving health care costs stem from: a) the universal human desire for immortality, and b) funding considerations more relevant to the funding source than to health care. While these considerations vary between the public, private, and academic sectors, in that there are different priorities and different sorts of things are owed as debts, debts must be paid in all sectors.

Another way of saying the first point is that history doesn't always repeat itself. That point has been qualified to say that the second time is farce; I believe that it is possible to do things better if one can learn from the past. Santayana's precept ("Those who do not learn from the past are condemned to repeat it.") also allows for learning. Even chronicles of repeated mistakes (Tuckman, 1979; Kennedy, 1988) suggest the possibility of doing right where others have failed. Even when we don't learn from the past, it can often be seen that the growth of knowledge, not necessarily its use, is linear.

Now to look at the chapters in turn to apply the model.

What Is a Psychiatrist?

The cyclical phenomenon is alternately placing mentally ill people in hospitals and then taking them out again. The linear phenomena are the varying expansions of different sorts of knowledge. In Chapter 1, Langsley and Yager note that the rise of moral treatment was preceded by an era of asylums and custody, itself preceded by a noninstitutional phase, just as moral treatment was succeeded by a time of institutionalization—cycles that continue to the present. Thus, the notion of the first revolution is arguable and somewhat attenuates the community dimension of the third. The second revolution, growth in the psychological dimension starting with Freud and the notion of the unconscious, was indeed revolutionary. The "third" revolution, community treatment, I think was actually psychopharmacology, and linked to the fourth, growth of the neurosciences. Thus the four revolutions are assignable into the social, psychological, and biological dimensions of psychiatry, respectively.

We didn't learn from the success of moral treatment, just as it can be argued that we didn't learn what we should have about what made hospitals successful. In fact, it is harder to put knowledge into play in the social dimension of psychiatry than in other two. Granted that the psychological dimension requires accepting irrationality, at least one does not have to work much beyond the individual. It is very hard to practice community psychiatry without a *community*, and many of our urban communities are composed of more predators than a discharged patient can avoid. A recently discharged patient is about as welcome, and is likely to suffer the same fate, as an abandoned car. The hope for the social dimension lies in demonstrating the differential efficacy of the various modalities that compose it, perhaps also in the creation of controlled communities, such as the residential uses to which state hospital campuses are now being put. The consequence for the future is that the growth of biological knowledge is likely to outrace the other two dimensions for the foreseeable future. The psychological dimension is next likely to be affected, because it will be investigated as how biological changes are expressed.

Langsley and Yager shift to medicolegal and economic issues by invoking the increase in malpractice suits. Psychiatry has been spared compared to the rest of medicine and psychiatric incomes are smaller targets of opportunity. Rapport tends to be better, patient reality-testing difficulties notwithstanding, and there are fewer procedures that can go wrong. The liability crisis is partly the growth of the legal profession and the tendency of juries to give more and larger awards. Is the growth of malpractice suits linear or cyclical? Being predominantly a social phenomenon, it is likely to be cyclical. However, the growth in the numbers of lawyers and laws is linear, so the pendulum is unlikely to swing very far back for some time. Psychiatric discipline actions are partly reactive and partly what a true profession should be doing—using its special knowledge to correct the mistakes of its practitioners. Psychiatric peer review organizations (PROs) are part of a general movement in medicine to pull back from unrestricted fee-for-service practices. In fact, psychiatry didn't drive costs up as far or as quickly as the other medical specialties, except in the few highly visible locales where there was adequate coverage to exploit. Recertification and licensure reregistration will be costly and are most likely to be driven by a desire to restrict the number of practicing physicians. The drive to look at outcome should be welcomed. For all its faults, the diagnosis related group (DRG) method of payment at least focuses on what is most important: does the patient get better?

Emphasis on competition seems to be waning as the marketing costs involved are perceived to add to health care costs without benefitting patients. Problems of managed care arrangements are discussed at length in comments on Chapter 2. There are inherent structural weaknesses in the health maintenance organization model. It is not clear whether the change of limited coverage for psychiatric illness is seen as a change up, from none to limited, or down, from more-than-limited to limited. In fact, the requirement for coverage has been increasing, mostly via state legislation, and the amount has had a boost in Medicare, at a time when Medicare was being reduced otherwise. Legislated coverage requirements often do not give primacy to psychiatrists, raising more issues of competition at the same time that coalitions of providers are required to work together to get the legislation passed.

Psychotherapy is a bridging issue between economics and the definition of psychiatry. By definition it is an area in which psychiatry is not likely to prevail (although remaining a contender) because it represents the psychological dimension only. Psychiatry is an entity that integrates biological, psychological, and social dimensions, but it cannot exist uniquely in any one of those dimensions.

The proposed definitions of a psychiatrist should take positive note of the emergence of certification by the American Board of Psychiatry and Neurology as a standard. Gone are the days when some training programs held themselves up as having higher standards than board certification could ever hope to imply. Remedicalization and the changing patterns of psychiatric practice are welcome consequences of the linear phenomenon of the growth of biological knowledge.

The most hopeful sign of a consensus in the definition of a psychiatrist has been the increasing similarity among the core material covered by residency programs and the narrowing of the range of orientations reported on surveys and in the various editions of the Directory of Psychiatric Residency Training Programs (Robinowitz et al., 1988). Another reassuring point about the data presented from surveys is that repeated surveys, while not comparable in many respects, probably show an enlarging definition of a psychiatrist. At least the specialty isn't restricting itself as much as in the times when competence in the subject areas now proposed as subspecialties in this volume weren't part of most core definitions. The Langsley and Yager repetition of their previous survey (see Chapter 1) does have the great advantage of comparability, although the addition of 26 new knowledge and skill items demonstrates growth. It is unfortunate that devising a treatment plan received less high rankings, as it has become a focus of accreditors, third-party payers, and other overseers. Many institutions require a psychiatrist's signature on the treatment plan, an unexploited opportunity to exert psychiatric leadership.

As one who works in the undersupplied public sector, I disagree with the notion that too many psychiatrists are being trained. Some of this thinking is related to the overall surpluses predicted by the Graduate Education National Advisory Committee, a conclusion challenged by several authorities (Schmeck, 1988), the lack of physician income decline (Mayer, 1987a; Page, 1987), and the news that 58 percent of the nation's 6600 hospitals are still actively recruiting physicians (Horowitz, 1988). Psychiatry is in there with guarantees of $84,000 to $125,000 net income (Pinkney, 1988). Child psychiatry continues to have a recruitment problem, to be the subject of a national conference in January 1989. There aren't enough physician researchers, and psychiatry and child psychiatry were found to be in greatest need by the

Graduate Medical Education National Advisory Committee (GMENAC; Plaut and Enzer, 1981), a report whose overall prediction of surplus is now being challenged (Schmeck, 1988). Granted, the terms and conditions of employment must be improved in these areas, but a greater supply is still needed to provide grist for the recruitment mill.

Langsley and Yager closed Chapter 1 with a comment about the inevitability of subspecialization: Because it is driven by the linear phenomenon of the growth of new knowledge, it most likely is inevitable. But a caveat should be sounded regarding its social and organizational dimension. American physicians were 85 percent specialized when public demand for primary care prevailed, and family practice, general internal medicine, and pediatrics have mushroomed. So far the public has not completed the reimbursement work needed to raise these specialties from being the lowest paid of all (yes, below psychiatry), but it is probably only a matter of time before this is done. Thus the proportion of specialists (subspecialists?) may be cyclical. Will there be subspecialties if no one will pay for them?

How Will the New Practice Settings Change Psychiatry?

In Chapter 2, Jonathan Borus uses Lester Thurow's notion of a three-tiered system: 1) "safety net," 2) have insurance enough to be above the net, and 3) have enough money to pay out of pocket to have what you really want. I agree, we have the three tiers already. The rest of the discussion deals mostly with the middle tier; many caveats must be voiced on behalf of the other two tiers.

The public sector operates in an unilluminating glow of rosy rhetoric while often being incapable of the simplest transaction, whether it is paying efficiently for fingerprinting its workers in New York or not opening the physician's mail in Michigan. Some practices in public psychiatry, such as paying an outside specialist $50 for three hours clinic work in New York, would be charming anachronisms if they were not so destructive to patient health. However, the rhetoric is not isolated from the political will of the people. Varyingly expressed wills have led to wide variations in public health spending (Medicaid in Mississippi is $400/person/year, but $3200/person/year in New York), especially eligibility, covered services, availability of physicians and nursing home services, quality of care, and reimbursement (Kimball, 1988a).

While it is difficult to generalize about what the public wants, it seems they want public institutions accredited, and the standards of accreditation are the same for public or private institutions. The people want better care for the homeless mentally ill, mentally ill criminal offenders, adolescent suicide attempters, and others, and they are likely to provide the resources to do so. Accreditation standards are also shifting to a single definition of a hospital as the Joint Commission of the Accreditation of Health Organizations (JCAHO) will be using the Accreditation Manual for Hospitals to evaluate psychiatric hospitals formerly visited under the Consolidated Standards. The Accreditation Manual for Hospitals standards require a medical rather than a professional staff, another opportunity for psychiatric leadership.

The out-of-pocket tier is where many psychiatrists have always been. Only in some military and governmental communities has coverage been adequate, and psychoanalysis has grown and matured without insurance coverage. Thus the demise of solo medical practice may not yet be at hand.

The projected growth of the "supermed" systems assumes an economy of scale and efficiency of operation that has not yet been demonstrated. Health care costs, driven by the desire to live as long as possible, if not forever, have surged (Kimball, 1988b). Some have suggested that realistic rationing, not promises of more efficiency, is the only solution to rising costs (Schwartz and Aaron, 1988). Mental health costs have surged as well (Freudenheim, 1987a), but they remain below the rates of other specialty care. There is not just a physician shortage, but a shortage of all types of labor (Pinkney, 1987). Insurance plans are in trouble (Kramon, 1988; Mullen, 1988; Southwick, 1987a). Hospital chains are shedding inefficient hospitals, the link to insurance not having worked out so well, but psychiatric hospitals are booming (Freudenheim, 1987b).

In this setting, managed care looked good because it could promise lower rates. But these rates are largely the function of having a young, healthy, employed insured group; as they age and retire, their utilization skyrockets. The mental health coverage issue is further beviled by a small group of high users. Whichever plan has them will cost more; the same coverage can be offered for much less by another plan because it doesn't have the high users. When they join and charge their expenses to the plan, the rates go up, just as if all of the heavy people had shifted to the other side of the boat. But health maintenance organizations in general are in trouble. Enrollments are less than expected (Freudenheim, 1988; Horowitz, 1988) or are no longer required (Mayer, 1987b). Half of all health maintenance organizations lost money in 1986 (Southwick, 1987b). Plans are closing in some areas (Meyer, 1987) and are having a rough time in others (Kenkel, 1987; Meyer, 1988; Wallace, 1987). Several factors work against such plans, especially those based in the work setting. They start with healthy young workers. Illness increases with age and markedly with retirement. The population inevitably moves into the latter conditions and the result is higher costs. At the same time, the venture capital used to start the organization must be paid off (remember the model is that all debts must be paid). In comes "competition," in that an open season for employee choice of insurance plans or care arrangements will inevitably result in new plans (again consisting of healthy young workers) offering better rates. Yet someone, probably the government, will have to bail out the old plans as they go bankrupt. Otherwise there will be slippage back to the safety net tier, where the government has to pay through Medicare or Medicaid.

There are indeed likely to be more constraints on physicians. The government will want to pay less per procedure, and it will ratchet down the diagnosis related groups. Profits will be squeezed, but the main effect will be to compress that middle tier. The insurance tier will be resilient. Even after years of trying, the 1 January 1988 jump in health insurance premiums was

10 percent to 70 percent, with the norm falling between 12 percent and 25 percent. Medicare, covering 31 million elderly and disabled Americans, raised its premiums 38 percent (Kramon, 1988). How come? Outpatient costs and ageing-in are major factors, plus more coverage, higher priced technology, and continued use of physicians despite efforts to limit visits. Out-of-pocket costs will be regarded as discretionary, seeing a psychiatrists as an alternative to cosmetic surgery, vacationing, and so forth. Here, the size of the tier is dictated more by the size of the national fortune than government interference. The deprofessionalization of medicine, already eloquently bewailed (Reed and Evans, 1987), is likely to be less of a problem in the out-of-pocket tier and will keep physicians there for a long time.

The impact of these changes on psychiatrists is arguable. More psychiatrists are likely to be needed in the public (safety net) tier, where staffing standards have arrived to show that hundreds, and probably thousands, are needed. Many states are mounting recruitment initiatives. Yes, other mental health professions pose competitive challenges, and psychotherapy (see above) is not the battleground on which to fight. But taking care of seriously mentally ill people, the high calling to which Yager and Langsley point out much psychiatric practice has shifted, will absorb many more practitioners than it presently has.

Much will depend on whether the psychiatrist, as reducer of other medical costs, retains credibility (Mumford et al., 1984; Taintor et al., 1984). The proposed list of interventions, for example, efficient brief psychotherapy, seems desirable; the systems constraints do not. Will systems really use gatekeepers if they aren't good at making diagnoses? Put another way, will the need to ration care overcome the fear of malpractice? How many suicides will be needed to give the psychiatrist access to the patients who should be seen? The research recommendations should be supported strongly.

The Future Psychiatrist as a Generalist: Arguments Against Credentialing Specialists

In Chapter 3, Sidney Weissman and Phillip Bashook argue eloquently for their four main points. Yes, the boundaries of medical specialties and subspecialties will continue to shift, but there will be boundaries to shift. Yes, there are problems defining the boundaries and basic core knowledge skills of a psychiatrist, but the Langsley and Yager studies show a high degree of consensus, just as did the Thompson and colleagues (1982) studies of training directors. While all residencies are not identical, the prevailing wail in the field is that they seem to be in danger of becoming so.

The argument of analogy with internal medicine is an interesting one because it serves both sides of the question. Against subspecialization is what has happened to internal medicine recently. Public frustration with the subspecialization of internal medicine was probably the major contributor to the drive for family medicine and general internal medicine. The notion that internal medicine has been doing well as a result of subspecialization certainly would be rejected by many public policy makers and health consumer groups. For more than a decade federal training monies have been flowing to primary care specialties. In effect, internal medicine defined its way out of the market, and the internal medical subspecialties no longer have the gatekeeping function. Psychiatry must be careful not to do the same thing; the absence of consideration of public attitudes and the flip side of economic arguments is cause for concern that we may not have based the discussions broadly enough.

For subspecialization, by analogy with internal medicine, is the prime driving force behind all subspecialization: the growth of knowledge and the recognition of the need for expertise. Nephrologists and cardiologists came into being because it was hard to maintain universal expertise in all aspects of internal medicine, and the public wanted to be in the most expert hands possible.

Weissman and Bashook close with a general systems theory approach to psychiatry that comes closest to my own preferred definition of psychiatry: that specialty of medicine that diagnoses and treats psychiatric disorders by integrating biological, psychological, and social knowledge and frames of reference. However, the argument doesn't defeat subspecialization. In fact it answers my second objection above: that the core of psychiatry hasn't been defined.

Subspecialization in Psychiatry: Positive, Negative, and Inevitable Aspects

Continuing the concern about with whom the subspecialization dialogue is being conducted, the Yager tendency to generalize from colleague's requests in Los Angeles can be countered by noting that the public and primary care gatekeepers do not have the fine-grained sensitivities he describes. The Yankelovich and other surveys show the public as having difficulty keeping in mind the difference between a psychologist and a psychiatrist. Outside of a few well-supplied metropolitan areas, the request is usually just for a "good psychiatrist." Considering that two-thirds of United States counties have no psychiatrist, the request is sometimes just for a psychiatrist. The primary care gatekeepers, often accused of using nonpsychiatrists, have not been pressing for subspecialization.

The issue of competition as a cause of subspecialization must take into account marketplace desires. The Jackie Mason joke about how the physician did in kidney in medical school reflects the health-conscious sophisticated-patient sort of concern with getting the most expert physician possible. Health policy makers have been demonstrating different concerns: how to get adequate low-cost primary care to everyone. If competition to do *that* becomes the highest priority, competition will work against subspecialization.

The purely professional arguments for subspecialization are persuasive; the professional concerns about what might happen are similarly well put. The greatest concern should be added cost of care and medical education. The least-likely-to-happen concern is the weakening of the core specialty, since that hasn't happened with child psychiatry. It isn't clear whether the added qualifications tier will be something to which the public will relate well. Certainly restrictive practice reimbursements may appear. The first step would be to follow the Canadian model of higher reimbursements for certain services, if performed by a specialist. This step would break the conceptual barrier presently hobbling the American insurance industry, which reimburses at the same rate for a procedural code regardless of who does it. The result would not necessarily be bad for psychiatry, because it could ease competition from nonpsychiatrists.

The educational implications are felicitous and seem to be the way most residency programs with the necessary resources are in fact functioning.

The Future of Consultation–Liaison Psychiatry as a Psychiatric Subspecialty

The setting versus psychiatrist roles grid is a good idea, and the general conclusion about subspecialization is agreeable. The first problem is that the settings and people (both patients and physicians) may overlap. The differing experiences of psychiatrists will inevitably lead to some having more experience at this than others. Some will become de facto subspecialists, the same way that Langsley and Yager propose that others have already become so—being known as being good at it, knowing more, doing more, and so on. After a while, they will probably seek some recognition of their superior knowledge, skills, and experience, and a self-certifying group may emerge. Houpt's assumptions can be taken as arguments as to why this may not happen; I will examine each in turn.

Money Will Drive the System

As noted in the discussion on Chapter 2, the proliferation of managed care settings may not continue. I believe that the system is driven by a desire to live forever, or at least as long as possible. Other people are usually far less willing to pay for this proclivity than one's loved ones or one is oneself, but they will still want to recruit good workers for General Motors and they may use health insurance coverage as a way of doing so. It is interesting to note how short-lived efforts to control costs have proved to be. Remember when it was thought there were enough nursing schools and nurses? Remember the Carter Administration's view of physicians as generators of health care costs and the Graduate Medical Education Committee's view of an oversupply of physicians? It was thought that New York City had too many hospital beds and many were closed; now there are thought to be too few and many more are being opened—a trend well underway before the acquired immunodeficiency syndrome (AIDS) appeared (Meyer, 1988).

Consultation–Liaison Psychiatry

Regarding "traditional consultation–liaison functions" not being able to fund themselves, Houpt takes a stand that varies from both sides in the recent debate about liaison psychiatry, in which it was agreed that consultation was doing fine, just liaison was in trouble. Yet each wave of demonstration funding seems to leave a little more liaison funding in place as the wave recedes down the shore. What has emerged is that there is much more grist for the consultation mill than was originally thought. The liaison assumption that others are ready, willing, and able to do the psychiatrist's work has not been proved on any one of those three points. Indeed, liaison psychiatry is like the trapeze artist falling because he can neither reach the consultation hold (since good liaison was held to reduce the need for consultations) nor go back to the liaison bar (his grant having run out).

In the midst of the drive to reduce the number of consultations, insufficient attention was paid to the following questions: What are the rates of medical and psychiatric illness in the general population? What are the loci of care for the general population? Among the loci of care, what is the rate of alcohol, drug, and mental illness in the general hospital population? What can the primary care physician, properly trained, do? What can be done by other health and mental health providers? What is left, in addition to teaching and research, for only the psychiatrist to do?

Only recently have data been derived that can help answer the question of the numbers of people and sorts of problems that a consultant should see or primary care physicians should be trained to help. Significant psychiatric morbidity resides in the community and in patients in the general health sector. Regier and his coworkers (1984) describe from the Epidemiologic Catchment Area (ECA) survey that 19 percent of adults in the United States have major psychiatric morbidity in any six-month period, while manifesting the following disorders: anxiety (8.3%), affective (6%), alcoholism (5%), drug abuse (2%). These alcohol, drug abuse, and mental disorders result in significant disability, costs, and deaths. For the year 1983, alcohol, drug abuse, and mental disorders cost $50.4 billion in direct and $200 billion in indirect treatment. The alcohol, drug abuse, and mental health illnesses were felt to be responsible for at least 1000 deaths per year: 69,000 alcohol-related deaths, including automobile accidents; 6000 deaths associated with drugs, and 33,000 deaths related to other mental health disorders.

With regard to alcohol, drug abuse, and mental health disorders in the general health sector, it has been estimated that up to 50 percent of all hospitalized patients exhibit significant psychological dysfunction, either as a result of or in conjunction with their medical/surgical disorder. (It must be taken into account that the majority of these studies are based on Diagnostic and Statistical Manual of Mental Disorders, second edition (DSM-II) criteria, and at least 15 percent to 20 percent of patients who are seen in the ambulatory medical setting have psychological dysfunction, either primary in nature or secondary to their physical illness. Sixty percent of Americans with alcohol and drug abuse disorders are seen exclusively in the general health sector. Regier and colleagues (1984) estimate that only 21 percent of these patients eventually obtain health care from mental health specialists. Consequently, even though 70 percent of patients with an alcohol or drug abuse disorder (in the previous 6 months) made at least one ambulatory medical visit, only 10 percent were examined by a mental health specialist. Finally, of the majority of patients with alcohol and drug abuse illnesses who received all of their care in the general medical sector, only 20 percent acknowledged that they were consulting the primary care physician for mental health reasons.

However, these epidemiologic data do not illuminate the difficulties primary care physicians have detecting mental disorders. Only 25 percent to 50 percent of patients with major depression tend to be identified by the primary care physician. Similarly, Jacobs and colleagues (1977) and others found that cognitive deficits were frequently overlooked by physicians. And the majority of patients in the general health sector with alcohol problems remain unidentified. Houpt opens a new vista by suggesting a greater amount of direct care responsibility for patients with medical psychiatric comorbidity. Physicians providing such services may well be at least de facto subspecialists.

It is not clear that level-of-care distinctions will necessarily become sharper. Certainly outpatient care, one such level, is less compelling because of new doubts about whether or not it is less expensive after all. Finding patients in psychiatric hospitals who supposedly could receive adequate care in nursing homes or community residences has become old hat. And the spread of technology can work both ways. The availability of low-cost machines for monitoring blood sugar levels leads to more outpatients. Lithotripsy for cholelithiasis will move such patients into hospitals that have the machines. But such hospitals may not be "tertiary." In fact, there seems to be a political tendency to spread the wealth: here a burn unit, there some transplants, there some other transplants, there a high-risk pregnancy and delivery program, there a hand microsurgery team, and so forth. The only thing of which to be sure is that there is more technology than people who know how to use it, keeping us with the basic explosion-of-knowledge rationale for subspecialization.

Houpt's suggested demographics of the future seem very likely to me; only more handicapped with high-tech prostheses should be added. They too will likely have some medical-psychiatric comorbidity.

The Predictions

The primary care outpatient sector may well be where some of the medically oriented psychiatrists are doing their work, since patients should be treated close to home. Because the psychiatrists are there, they may be used for consultation and liaison. It is true that there is little at present, but that doesn't mean there will necessarily be less.

Within the community hospital it is not clear that neuropsychologists will necessarily move from assessment into providing treatment; most haven't so far. Liaison teaching in the general hospital will depend on marketing and psychiatry's ability to maintain a presence. Within the tertiary hospital, it is agreed that general psychiatric consultation should be within the competence of all psychiatrists, although de facto subspecialization is to be expected. The modest subspecialization recommended for medical-psychiatric units is desirable, and the continuance of psychotherapy is agreeable. In all of the settings involved, the self-referral or patient-referral influence must be considered. As the mental illness model, patient education, and destigmatization gain, there will probably be more self-referral.

The route to the proposed specialization favors psychiatry-cum-fellowship, rather than passing two board-certifying examinations. This seems to be a good way to ensure that the turf involved remains psychiatric, but the attractions of dual board certification will be very great.

The Future of Psychiatric Education

There is little to add to Jerald Kay's and Alan Tasman's definitive review of the field, except doubts already expressed in discussing other chapters. Will there really be a surplus of physicians? If so, why don't we see it, now less than two years from surplus time? Why aren't market forces operating to reduce prices if supply is up? Doesn't the emergence of corporate medicine indicate that at least some players believe that there is money to be made. Yet how can money be made by adding more salaries to be paid? Kay and Tasman suggest one point to complement the following chapter by adding computers and informatics to the cutting edge. Indeed, the use of computers illustrates the subspecialization explosion-of-knowledge paradigm. Now there is almost too much to be learned about patients. References on their maladies can be obtained in the flicker of a cathode ray tube. Past laboratory data, past history, all previous medications, et cetera, can be summoned up more quickly than they can be evaluated. Part of the information explosion is the availability of cost data, and we shall be teaching much more about cost management than before.

The Cutting Edge: A Blueprint for Curriculum Change and Future Research in Psychiatry

There is no argument to be had with any item in this chapter. One could quibble regarding whether this or that was truly more significant than something else, but more time would have to pass before data for such arguments could be brought to bear against a well-designed and well-executed survey such as this. Instead, one can add and face the problems of subtraction. The additions have already been made by Kay and Tasman; no subtractions are proposed, probably because to do so would be to weaken the case for subspecialization. What is likely to be the result? Probably three years of core training and two years of subspecialty fellowship, or residency for a total of five.

Summary

The previous papers are diverse in their fatalism or willingness to buck the future by trying to do something about it. Clearly the attempts should be made to influence the future favorably. In this respect, our main allies are the patient and family groups that have mushroomed recently. They will grow and prosper whether or not psychiatry helps them, but both can do much better with mutual assistance. The agenda should include a workable illness model and a workable biopsychosocial model with which to attack illness, patient, family, and public education; destigmatization; research; and other influential factors.

We must take the profit takers with a grain of salt. Quick profit is inconsistent with long-term commitment. Venture capitalists are in to make a deal, clear a profit, and get out. Adding layers of management and bureaucracy will not necessarily be financeable through some economies of scale, such as mass purchasing or rationing of services, like limiting access.

References

Freudenheim M: Mental health costs surge. New York Times, p D2, 1 Dec 1987a

Freudenheim M: Specialty health care booms. New York Times, pp D1, D5, 15 Dec 1987b

Freudenheim M: Prepaid programs for health care encounter snags. New York Times, pp 1, 34, 31 Jan 1988

Horowitz MG: IPAs flounder in New York City. Health Week 1(8):1, 42, 23 Nov 1987

Horowitz MG: Hospitals offer guarantees in recruiting MDs. Health Week 2(1):6, 36, 4 Jan 1988

Jacobs J, Bernhard MR, Delgado A, et al: Screening for organic mental syndrome in the medically ill. Ann Intern Med 1977; 86:40–46

Kenkel PJ: Competition and slowed enrollment hurt managed care companies—study. Modern Healthcare pp 58–60, 20 Nov 1987

Kennedy P: The Rise and Fall of Great Powers. New York, Random House, 1988

Kimball MC: Big differences among states in Medicaid spending. Health Week 2(1):3, 36, 4 Jan 1988a

Kimball MC: Nation's health care bill to hit $544 billion in 1988. Health Week 2(3):8, 19 Jan 1988b

Kramon G: Insurance costs for health care rise sharply. New York Times, pp 1, D5, 12 Jan 1988

Mayer D: Lockheed ends first-ever program requiring 1-year HMO enrollment. Health Week 1(8):1, 23 Nov 1987a

Mayer D: Consumer advocates blast big jump in 1986 physician income. Health Week 1(8):36, 7 Dec 1987b

Mayer D: Cramped NYC hospitals to get up to 500 beds. Health Week 2(1):1, 36, 4 Jan 1988

Meyer H: Plan closings net 3rd-quarter loss for HMO operator. American Medical News p 5, 27 Nov 1987

Meyer H: HMOs, PPOs take beating, but keep ticking. American Medical News p 15, 1 Jan 1988

Mullen P: Blue Cross/Washington sees 54% rate hike. Health Week 2(1):1, 36, 4 Jan 1988

Mumford E, Schlesinger EJ, Glass GV, et al: A new look at evidence about reduced cost of medical utilization following mental health treatment. Am J Psychiatry 1984; 141:1145–1158

Page L: SMS survey: MDs earning more but working more hours, too. American Medical News, pp 13, 15, 20 Nov 1987

Pinkney D: Manpower crisis: growing labor shortage in all areas crippling hospitals across the nation. American Medical News, pp 1, 12, 20 Nov 1987

Pinkney D: More hospitals using financial incentives to lure MDs. American Medical News p 16, 19 Feb 1988

Plaut EA, Enzer NB: The GMENAC projection of a major shortage of psychiatrists by 1990. Journal of Psychiatric Education 1981; 5(4):346–355

Reed RR, Evans D: The deprofessionalization of medicine. JAMA 1987; 258:3279–3282

Regier DA, Myers JK, Kramer M, et al: The NIMH Epidemiologic Catchment Area (ECA) Program: historical context, major objectives, and study population characteristics. Arch Gen Psychiatry 1984; 41:934–941

Robinowitz C, Taintor Z, Kay J (eds): Directory of Psychiatry Training Programs, fourth edition. Washington, DC, American Psychiatric Press, Inc., 1988

Schmeck HM: Shortage of doctors viewed as likely by the end of the century. New York Times, p B5, 6 April 1988

Schwartz WB, Aaron HJ: A tough choice on health care costs. New York Times, Op-Ed page, 6 Apr 1988

Southwick K: Half of all HMOs are losing money. Health Week 1(4):1, 13, 28 Sep 1987a

Southwick K: Blue Cross of California slices deficits as big losses continue. Health Week 1(6):4, 37, 26 Oct 1987b

Taintor Z, Widem P, Barrets N (eds): Cost Considerations in Mental Health Treatment: Settings, Modalities, and Providers. NIMH, Mental Health Economics (#2), Rockville, MD, DHHS Publication No. (ADM) 84–1295, 1984

Thompson MGG, Henderson P, Bowden C, et al: Residency training priorities: international and child versus adult comparisons. Journal of Psychiatric Education 1982; 6:144–153

Tuckman, B: The March of Folly. New York, Random House, 1979

Wallace C: Two large HMOs report third quarter losses. Modern Healthcare, p 12, 20 Nov 1987

Chapter 10

A Futuristic View of Psychiatry

Joel Yager, M.D.

Prediction is a risky business: No one knows how to do it well, and certainly no one knows how to do it flawlessly. Yet, with psychiatry in constant flux, in order to anticipate and plan we are obliged to peer ahead as best we can. This chapter will introduce some of the principles and methods used by professional futurists, describe predictions that have been made for society and medicine as a whole for the next quarter century that may directly impact the practice of psychiatry and related professions, and discuss possible coping strategies for the profession.

Paradoxically, long-range predictions, on the order of several hundred years, and very short-range predictions, on the order of one or two, perhaps even five or ten years, may be easier to make accurately than are predictions in the middle range. For the far future, even simple extensions of contemporary technology permit us to envision great changes, provided we are not obliged to figure out the costs of such advances, or to state precisely the dates by which they will occur.

Futurists call our attention to several different types of events: the *likely,* based on what we know today and can easily extrapolate; the *possible,* based on optimistic extensions of current work and intuitive knowledge about technological breakthroughs we are likely to attain; and the *unexpected,* those serendipitous and unimagined findings that require an entirely new theory or worldview for explanation and that change some of the basic paradigms of our knowledge. In making predictions about the future, we must attend not only to those events and processes that encourage change, but also to those social and technological forces that retard discovery and constrain the implementation of change. Such inertial forces include economic and social value issues. These forces have all shaped the evolution of modern medicine and psychiatry up to the present, and will all be at work in their future evolution.

To provide some perspective about the rate of change in medicine, the bicentennial Clinical Pathological Case Conference of the New England Journal of Medicine (Majno et al., 1976) is informative. Case number one, admitted to the Massachusetts General Hospital in 1821, less than 200 years ago, was a patient in his 20s who had a hospital course of about six months between his admission and death in the hospital from syphilis and diarrhea.

135

He was treated with a variety of medications, each of which probably added to his discomfort, if not actually hastening his demise. The few effective drugs in the pharmacopeia at that time included opium, ipecac, Peruvian bark for malaria, citrus fruit for scurvy, and foxglove. Other medications were either placebos or were actively detrimental to health. Imagine the situation of a physician in those days: there was no germ theory of disease, no notion of antisepsis for surgery, no effective antibiotic. The existence of x-rays were not only unknown, they were wholly unimagined. Electronics were unknown; indeed, knowledge about electricity was primitive. Chemistry was in its infancy, and the periodic table was not yet described. To have predicted anything close to modern medical science would have invited scorn. So you can imagine how incredulous Benjamin Rush and his students would be if they had the opportunity to see contemporary medicine, just as we would be incredulous if we were suddenly transported 200 years into the future via time-machine to witness medicine and psychiatry in 2190.

Perhaps we would be better prepared for such a journey if we studied Arthur C. Clarke's laws of the future. These three laws, set forth by a leading contemporary scientist and visionary—the creator of "2001: A Space Odyssey" and the prophet of the stationary orbit for satellites—can help us evaluate the myriad of predictions with which we're faced as *we* to try to peer 200 years ahead into the future. Clarke's Laws are as follows (Clarke, 1972, pp. 129–130):

1. When a distinguished but elderly scientist says that something is possible, he is almost certainly right. When he states that something is impossible, he is very probably wrong.

2. The only way to discover the limits of the possible is to go beyond them into the impossible.

3. Any sufficiently advanced technology is indistinguishable from magic.

Clarke points out that the third law, scientific technology seeming like magic, is not always due to complexity. Sometimes the most important thing about a new idea is simply that it forces us to look at the obvious in a new, unanticipated way. In an essay entitled "Hazards of Prophecy," Clarke has compiled a list of advances, some of which were (or have been) expected, either on the basis of then current technology or general fancy, and others that were totally unanticipated (Clarke, 1972). The expected, not all of which have as yet come to pass, included automobiles, flying machines, steam engines, submarines, spaceships, telephones, robots, death rays, transmutation of matter, artificial life, immortality, invisibility, levitation, teleportation, communication with the dead, observing the past and future, and telepathy.

Among the unexpected, those advances that caught the scientific community completely by surprise, were x-rays, nuclear energy, radio and television, electronics, photography, sound recording, quantum mechanics, relativity, transistors, lasers, masers, superconductors, superfluids, atomic clocks, determining the composition of celestial bodies, dating the past (as with carbon-14), detecting invisible planets, the ionosphere, and the Van Allen radiation belts. Thus, the history of the past 200 years cautions us that the future will consist of much more than simple extensions of the expected; it will probably contain healthy doses of the unexpected as well.

Methods for Predicting the Future

A variety of methods for thinking about the future have been described, and several have been applied to areas that impact on psychiatry's future. Comprehensive forecasting must take into account changes in technology, economics, values and other aspects of society. Seminal thinkers in this area have included Herman Kahn (Kahn and Weiner, 1969; Kahn et al., 1976), Daniel Bell (Bell, 1968), and Alvin Toffler, who through such books as *Future Shock* (Toffler, 1970), *The Futurists* (Toffler, 1973), and others (Toffler, 1974, 1980, 1983) did much to inform the public at large about these concepts. Parenthetically, Toffler's expressions of gratitude to the psychiatrist Dr. Donald Klein for his comments on early drafts of *Future Shock* and *The Third Wave* indicate that some psychiatric thought may have already had significant influence on popular thinking about the future.

The following discussion of methods for the study of the future is compiled from material presented by Toffler (1970, 1973), Gordon (1972), Jungk (1970), Waskow (1972), Renfro (1987), and others. Full application of futurist methods requires appraising all available sources of current information about the problems under review (an intelligence unit), methods for thinking through all the alternatives (a modeling unit), and feedback and research units to assess the impact of the imagined alternatives on various consumers of the future. Several of these methods are often applied concurrently.

Genius Forecasting is a method relying on the genius and insights of the forecaster, and heavily on luck. *Trend Extrapolation* involves forecasts made on the basis of straight-line extensions of demographics, technological developments with obvious implications, applications not yet effected, and even the likely adoption of new health and welfare programs based on their appearance in other Western countries, particularly Scandinavia. These forecasts are best made with respect to "high inertia" systems, that is, things embedded in the economy. This method's major weakness is the assumption that forces at work in the past will probably continue to be at work in the future. Nevertheless, many of today's most successful futurists, such as John Naisbitt, author of *Megatrends* (Naisbitt, 1984), attempt to detect early trends through extensive and informed reading of national and international trade magazines and newspapers, as the basis for extensions (Naisbett, 1985).

Consensus Methods include brainstorming, discussion groups, and the Delphi technique (Gordon, 1972), and these are the most commonly used methods for predicting the future. Brainstorming can be technically and even mechanically assisted, using group creativity techniques such as Synectics

(Gordon, 1961) and the computer-assisted generation of alternative possibilities. The Delphi technique involves the circulation of anonymously authored opinions about likely futures for comment and revision among a group of experts. Elimination of the social prestige and influence that would occur in response to the original authors' identities decreases the subsequent biases of the reviewers, and the resulting predictions, generated from several iterations of these opinions, are often more accurate than those resulting from face-to-face discussion.

Simulation Methods are many, although few have been applied to psychiatry's future. These include 1) Mechanical analogues, of which wind tunnels to predict performance during development of airplanes and cars are an example; 2) Mathematical analogues include a set of equations, e.g., describing the economic situation of a country or the distribution of specialties and geographic locations of medical school graduates in relation to other demographic factors; 3) Metaphorical analogues can be exemplified by the growth of bacteria in a colony taken to depict human population growth or medical specialty saturation in a geographic area; and 4) Games analogues, e.g., interactions between two or more players in carefully contrived laboratory games taken to represent or predict social interactions in the real world (from a psychiatric perspective, these methods have been used in research studies of family processes and of small group interactions).

Simulation games usually have the following five elements: 1) rules of play to govern the interaction among players and other variables in the game; 2) objectives or goals, where players must work cooperatively toward a joint goal (non-zero sum games) or competitively toward goals which cannot be shared (zero-sum games); a single game may have elements of both; 3) a method of translating the moves of the players into indicators which measure the degree of attainment of goals (this device may be a game board, a mathematical model, or another group of participants charged with the responsibility of judging the effect of the players' moves); 4) a display system to illustrate the progress of the game; and 5) a set of exogenous variables to introduce "outside events" into the play.

Cross-impact Matrix Methods involve estimations of the likelihood of event B occurring if event A occurs. Groups of possible independent variables are set out in various combinations, and the effects of these on the subsequent behavior of other groups of dependent variables are assessed.

Scenario Building takes into account that scenarios describe future histories; they are not predictive devices, but simply devices to stimulate thought. Scenarios built for health and mental health field predictions commonly include titles such as *status quo, hard times, increased resources,* and *transformation* (Council on Long Range Planning and Development, 1987). Several types are described, including: 1) Surprise-free projections: these "standard worlds" are, according to Kahn and Weiner, unlikely, because the future always contains surprises; and 2) Canonical variations: in these scenarios a standard world is imagined, but something unexpected is injected into it at some point.

Recent computer simulation methods combining cross-matrix analysis and scenario building have been applied to the health field. Probabilities for each of a large number of events, such as government funding policies, are estimated by a group of experts in the health field (informed speculation) and the computer cranks out various complex scenarios with probability estimates. Low probability events (those with less than 1 in 10 chances of occurring) are included, because, if more than 10 percent of these are present in a given scenario, at least one is likely to happen (Renfro, 1987).

Decision Trees are graphic devices that demonstrate alternative approaches to critical decisions.

The systematic study of history for relevant analogies has been proposed as a potentially useful method for generating options for the present and future. For example, we can review the considerations undertaken by decision makers during past crises, examine the consequences of their actual choices, and attempt to assess the pertinence of their situations to those that currently face us (Toffler, 1970, 1973).

Creative Disorder is a method used by groups of people that Waskow has called *participatory futurists* that consists of attempts to project workable visions of the future over a one-generational time period and then attempts to build chunks of that future in the present (Waskow, 1972). However, these attempts are not generally done with the help of powerful societal institutions, but rather from the grassroots level, from the bottom up, without the permission of the powerful and often against the laws or moves of the present order. Such work includes unorthodox projects, such as neighborhood level quasigovernments in metropolitan centers. Waskow suggests that society should establish future gaming centers with living attempts to create alternative types of schools, neighborhoods, and other social institutions. Arcosanti, an experiment in the Arizona desert, is an example, as are R.D. Lainge's non-institutional alternatives for psychotic patients in Britain. Toffler's *intentional community,* a utopian idea, is a related concept; for example, Toffler (1980) suggests the creation of group medical practices that take advantage of the latest medical technology, but whose members accept modest pay and pool their profits to run completely new styles of medical schools.

Several technological tools that would be extremely valuable to futuristic research in psychiatry are not yet available. Toffler cites the need for generally agreed upon *social indicators,* analogous to economic indicators, to enable us to better measure the quality of life and the level of transience in society (Toffler, 1972, p. 104). We also need a general model of value change, but none has yet been developed. We see that values change, and seem to be changing with increasing rapidity, shaped by pressures of technology, such as birth control devices, advertising, the mass media, economic conditions, and so-forth, and that these changes seem to affect psychological well being and perhaps psychiatric morbidity. Powerful and rapidly shifting economic forces appear to be exceptionally important determinants of who in society works in what types of jobs; how such efforts are distributed in families; how, when, and why traditional family and social roles break down; why families break up, and other events that have major psychiatric importance (Harris, 1981). Finally, additional research is needed into better methods for predicting the future, and for using operations research methods to actually shape the future.

Futurists' Predictions That Carry Implications for Psychiatry and Other Mental Health Professions

Attracted by the coming millennium, over the past decades futurists have been busily generating scenarios and lists of predictions as to what the future will hold for us. Many of these "big picture" predictions carry important implications for psychiatry, so that before focusing on psychiatry per se, it may be helpful to review some of these broader visions of the future. In a 1967 paper entitled "The Next Thirty-three Years: a Framework for Speculation," Kahn and Weiner (1969) provided *surprise-free projections* for the future of the century.

According to these authors, the world will become increasingly sensate, empirical, this-worldly, humanistic, pragmatic, and utilitarian. With an increased size of the leisure, white-collar, and middle classes, there may be an increase in the demand for psychotherapy services, a middle-class value. The world will also become more bourgeois, meritocratic, and bureaucratic, with worldwide industrialization, affluence, urbanization, literacy and education, decreasing the importance of primary and secondary professions and increasing the importance of the service professions. And the world will become increasingly rich in technological and scientific advancements. Overall, Kahn and Weiner listed 100 technical innovations likely to be developed between 1967 and the year 2000. My assessment is that about 40 of these would impact on the practice of the mental health professions.

Also in 1967, Olaf Helmer, codeveloper of the Delphi technique, listed those developments he forecast would be "virtually certain" by the year 2000, and those he considered to be "less probable" but which still had a good chance of being present (Helmer, 1967). Among those Helmer predicted to be "virtually certain" that would most likely impact psychiatry were: 1) The world gross national product will be more than three and possibly four times what it was in 1967. 2) People will live in urban complexes, surrounded by numerous automata. In particular there will be central data banks and libraries with fully automated access and, a full credit card economy. Highly sophisticated teaching machines will be in use. Portable videotelephones will facilitate communication among persons everywhere, and this process will be further enhanced by the availability of automated translation from one language to another. 3) Personality-affecting drugs will be as widely used and accepted as alcoholic beverages were in 1967. 4) The life spans of most people will be extended by replacing worn or diseased organs with artificial plastic and electronic organs. 5) Highly intelligent machines will act as effective collaborators with scientists and engineers.

According to Helmer's predictions, the following are *less* probable, but still have a good chance for being part of the world in the year 2000: 1) Cooperation between humans and machines may progress to the point of actual brain-computer synthesis, enabling humans to extend their intelligence by direct electromechanical interaction between the brain and a computing machine. 2) We may learn, through molecular engineering, to control hereditary defects and the aging process, and to induce the artificial growth of new limbs and organs. We may also have drugs that increase intelligence. Helmer further suggested that the next great breakthrough in the social sciences, comparable in significance to such physical breakthroughs as the creation of artificial life or the control of thermonuclear energy, may well be the construction of a theory of organizations that succeeds in dealing rationally with situations of interpersonal or international conflict.

Before putting too much faith into the predictions of these futurists, we should ask how accurate such predictions turn out to be. In rating a large study of expert predictions made in 1964 about what the world would be like in 1984, Calder (1984) found that on the average the predictions, based mostly on trend analysis, were "fair to good". Most problems in prediction were due to oversights, many of which were unavoidable. Many other erroneous fantasies were over-optimistic predictions based on developments that were in fact technologically possible, but which failed to consider economic problems of resource allocation that would have been necessary to implement some of these excellent ideas. Some of the best psychiatrically relevant predictions were based on S shaped curves, built on what were the new and emerging technologies, such as brain transplants and neuropeptides.

With this in mind, consider what futurists of the 1980s predict about areas that will impact on psychiatry:

In demographics, we can anticipate a drop in birth rate, increases in divorce and trial marriages, and an increase in the aging population and their "gray power" (Cetron and O'Toole, 1982). These trends are likely to result in more single-parent homes, shorter adolescences, and less of a *child-centered* society (Toffler, 1980). There will also be an increase in less skilled graduates, poorer education, and more drop outs (Naisbitt, 1984).

In social policy, we are likely to see some increase in social programs following the Swedish model, such as better child care and government-funded catastrophic health insurance (Cetron and O'Toole, 1982). However, because of cost pressures, we are not likely to see any major changes in discriminatory policies toward mental illness (Ginzberg, 1987).

In values, increasing *high technologies* will lead to a concurrent interest in *high touch,* that is, a need for basic human contact and a search for meaning, identity, and spirituality to attack the loneliness resulting from fragmentation and loss of the extended and even nuclear family (Toffler, 1980). More people will seek therapy (Ginzberg, 1987), and, although Toffler believes this will lead to a need for more psychiatrists to help provide a *life-organizing function* as *structure* providers (Toffler, 1980), this need could be fulfilled by other nonmedical therapists.

In technology, drugs may be available to enhance memory, cure alcoholism and drug addictions (Cetron and O'Toole, 1982), and reduce illness via gene splicing. Cetron and O'Toole (1982) also believe that, by the year 2050, the human life span may be 150 to 200 years, bringing along major shifts in how we mature, work, reproduce, plan ahead, and socialize. The psychiatric implications for such developments are enormous.

At the same time, the increasingly high cost of high-tech medical care will generate the need for low-tech alternatives, particularly for terminal and chronic care, such as hospices and less expensive asylums (Naisbitt, 1984).

The extensive availability of telecommunications and telenetworking will greatly influence how medicine is practiced, for example, on how expert consultation is obtained and employed (Toffler, 1980; Naisbitt, 1984). For psychiatry, teletherapy, teleconsultation, and the use of computer-assisted expert system programs as adjuncts to psychotherapy are likely to lead to new modes of practice (Maxmen 1978; Gould 1986).

In medical economics, forecasters examining the short-term environment have studied the changing environment in which medicine will be practiced. John Naisbitt and his group (1985) cite the following issues: cost containment leading to cost cutting, marketing, competition, and "Doc in the Box" forms of practice (that is, the interchangeable physician in walk-in, urgent-care settings); increasing subspecialty practices; and the use of computers in consultation. All of these in conjunction will lead to a slew of new ethical questions.

The Current Status of Psychiatry: Where Are We Now?

Despite the relatively rapid changes and indisputable advances in psychiatry over the past decades, particularly in basic science, psychopharmacology and even the beginnings of empirically validated psychotherapies and psychosocial interventions, psychiatric science is still in a relatively primitive state. Psychiatry is in the midst of controversy concerning diagnoses; how to distribute available resources among research and therapeutic efforts directed toward biological, psychological, family, and social systems; how to finance mental health care; and how to share responsibilities for mental health services with primary care physicians and nonmedical mental health providers.

We lack basic types of information, measurement tools, and concepts. We still know very little about etiology and pathogenesis at levels where valid diagnoses and rational treatments are possible; about the extent to which the availability of mental health practitioners affects such basic outcome measures as the rate of psychiatric casualties in suicide, homicide, and chronicity; and about the extent to which paraprofessionals, aided by modern technology, might be able to effectively carry out some roles now assigned to mental health professionals.

We need better data and more sophisticated models to describe relationships between types and intensities of treatment and outcome. We have not yet demonstrated relationships between the amount of professional time spent with patients (and how that time is spent) and therapeutic benefit, or even that treatment versus no treatment will usually produce improvement for certain disorders. For example, without much empirical evidence, many psychiatrists currently treat numerous disorders as if once-a-week therapy were an effective frequency for all these problems; this is undoubtedly related to insurance company benefits and patient ability to pay. We need better data to help shape practice models *and* insurance benefits in a more rational fashion.

Although many scientific advances are being made in basic fields and in some clinical areas as well, even what we know in theory has not been translated into practice. As Judd Marmor described in his 1976 American Psychiatric Association Presidential Address, unchanged in the interim, we are woefully behind many other countries when it comes to aftercare, posthospital planning, including provision of meaningful work, and life settings. Eastern European psychiatrists, for example, can much more easily manipulate patients' environments than can we.

Psychiatric practice is, for the most part, not yet scientific. According to Kuhn's (1962) criteria for judging scientific fields, psychiatry is probably in a prescientific state, a preparadigmatic state. In describing the prescientific, preparadigmatic world of physical optics before Newton, for example, Kuhn said the following (1962, p. 13):

> Though the field's practitioners were scientists, the net result of their activity was something less than science. Being able to take no common body of belief for granted, each writer on physical optics felt forced to build his field anew from its foundations. In doing so, his choice of supporting observations and experiment was relatively free, for there was no standard set of methods or of phenomena that every optical writer felt forced to employ or explain." Kuhn further stated (1962, p. 15), "and it remains an open question what parts of social science have yet acquired truly scientific paradigms at all.

According to Kuhn, a paradigm defines what the legitimate questions and methods are for a given field of inquiry. The established paradigm is the one accepted by the workers in a given area, and the available (and legitimized) methods determine the nature of research and the questions that may be asked. Although contemporary psychiatry puzzles about the same fascinating questions that have been around for eons (for example, the nature of consciousness, emotion, and thought and their relation to brain activity) and in spite of rapid and informative advances in neuroscience and cognitive psychology, we still seem far from being able to answer these questions in a meaningful or profound way. Our methods and concepts fall short, and, since we are unable to operationally define and quantitatively measure many of these phenomena, they have been judged in some circles as unworthy for scientific study at the present time, because the study of complex problems with useless tools and inadequate concepts usually produces useless data. In spite of rapid advances in brain imaging and neurophysiology, we are still not able to measure the subtle physics of large neural nets, or to image functional activities of the living brain in anything more than the crudest fashion. Advances in these areas will permit us to pose better questions not even conceived at present, just as each technological advance in chemistry, biochemistry, and genetics has helped shape the next set of ever more sophisticated research questions.

Kuhn (1962, p. 15) continues:

> In the absence of a paradigm or some candidate for a paradigm, all of the facts that could possibly pertain to the development of a given science are likely to seem equally relevant. As a result, early fact gathering is a far more nearly random activity than the one that subsequent scientific development makes familiar. Furthermore, in the absence of a reason for seeking some particular form of more recondite information, early fact-gathering is usually restricted to the wealth of the data that lie ready to hand.

And still later Kuhn states (1962, p. 47), "the pre-paradigm period, in particular, is regularly marked by frequent and deep debates over legitimate methods, problems and standards of solution, though these serve rather to define schools than to produce agreement."

Doesn't this sound familiar for psychiatry? Although some psychiatrists believe that they possess a workable paradigm, in biological psychiatry or psychoanalysis or behaviorism, or family systems, and that their Rosetta Stone is at hand, most readily admit to being in the premessianic, preparadigmatic state of knowing that far more powerful explanatory theories and models are required.

Futures Research in Psychiatry

Aside from *genius* forecasting, there has been little in the way of systematic research on psychiatry's future, although what has been produced is of interest. The Future Mental Health Services Project has generated a series of four scenarios for the year 2010, called status quo, increased resource, hard times, and transformation, based mostly on potential variations in social and economic forces, but with relatively little attention given to the potential impact of new knowledge (Institute for Alternative Futures, 1985). For each scenario, this group considered a large number of shaping conditions and ventured projections for such factors as the gross national product (GNP), the rate of growth of inflation, unemployment, family cohesiveness-divorce rates, the number of people on welfare, the number of people in public housing, the number of individuals below the poverty level, and the percentage of the gross national product devoted to health care systems and mental illness. Also considered were the extent of diagnosable mental illness; the position of the legal and jail systems regarding mental illness; the availability of services through primary care services; specialty mental health settings; various public and private hospitals; outpatient services and peer care; financing relationships among federal, state, and county governments and employers, insurance companies, and individuals; and the availability of all manner of professional, paraprofessional, and self-care personnel. The resulting scenarios are extrapolations based on the anticipated impacts of primarily financially driven limiting conditions. The transformation scenario, more fanciful than the others, presumes more dramatic value changes in society that lead to greater national interest in wellness and in healthier lifestyles as depicted through less substance abuse, more stress reduction practices, more exercise, better diets, and earlier interventions for health and mental health problems, particularly through employee assistance programs (EAPs) at the worksite.

Another organized "futures" activity has been spearheaded by John Talbott, M.D., through the American Psychiatric Association. In this project, four working groups produced stimulus documents to serve as the basis for larger group discussion and recommendations. The first two work groups to generate papers considered scientific advances and clinical services. These papers were fed into two other groups that considered their implications for funding and for education, and all four papers were discussed at a larger conference in December 1987.

One additional study, by Strauss et al. (1984), described in greater detail in Chapter 8, examined the predictions of psychiatric experts for the coming decade with respect to scientific advances.

In the absence of other systematic futuristic research in psychiatry, we turn to the intuitive, educated guesses of those psychiatric visionaries bold enough to publically pronounce what they see in their crystal balls. Some are more optimistic (Langsley, 1981; Pardes, 1979; Tarjan, 1984) and some are more pessimistic (Torrey, 1974; Clare, 1982); some concern themselves primarily with social and economic influences on psychiatry (Ginzburg, 1987; Beigel, 1986; Macdonald, 1987; Talbott, 1985a, 1985b), and others focus largely on the effects of possible scientific advances (Detre, 1987; Freedman, 1982; Eisenberg, 1973; Havens, 1986; West, 1973). Prominent among these figures are many recent presidents of the American Psychiatric Association, who have felt the need to prophesy for the profession in their presidential addresses. They may be excused if they waxed somewhat more optimistic than others, since the demand characteristics of the presidential speech may require "upbeat" messages (Lehman, 1985). However, many others worth considering have written without the benefit of a formal pulpit (Williams and Johnson, 1979; Maxmen, 1976; Detre, 1987; Eisenberg, 1972; Havens, 1986; West, 1973). We must also recognize that, to some extent, all of these visions must be taken with a grain of salt, and that, as Lehman (1986) has pointed out, the personality of the author probably plays a major role in the prophesies offered.

For the sake of simplicity, we can broadly divide this discussion into those futures shaped by social and economic issues, and those shaped by scientific advances.

Social and Economic Futures

In 1974, Alfred Freedman predicted that several major forces would shape psychiatry's future over the next several years; accountability, maldistribution of medical specialists, legitimacy for the legality of what we do, validating of our methods and operations, and further determination of the appropriate role of the psychiatrist. In the early and mid-1970s, he translated these issues into several expectations.

The first expectation held that, to the extent that we were paid by third-party payers, including the government, there was an obvious and already present movement (trend analysis) toward mandatory credentials with periodic recertification and toward quality assurance of practice. These activities were expected to occur before we really knew how to do them well. Now, 15 years later, we can see that only some of this has come to pass. Credentialing and periodic certification are still not mandatory, although both issues remain actively discussed and debated. Quality assurance activities and additional regulation, in hospital practice primarily, is certainly with us. And, as Freedman predicted, we are still unable to competently examine for competence, and we struggle with the problematic quality of quality assurance.

Secondly, a decade ago it was thought that the problem of maldistribution of physicians would be solved, within a few years, through federal mandate and marketplace forces. Some expected the establishment of a national residency board that would eventually regulate the number of medical school graduates to enter post graduate residency training in each medical specialty and in each geographic region. Although this has not yet come to pass, a new federally mandated Council on Graduate Medical Education has recently been established, and this group will undoubtedly continue to consider and give advice on these issues. Meanwhile, telecommunication methods and psychiatric "circuit riders" using airplanes may help provide services to remote areas.

A third expectation recognized that the legality and legitimacy of psychiatric activities would remain a rapidly changing area, and we can expect more ferment in the future regarding the right to treatment, confidentiality, informed consent, safeguards prior to the administration of psychiatric medication and ECT, and the conduct of psychiatric research on children, prisoners, and voluntary and involuntary adult patients.

The fourth expectation was that concerns regarding the validity of our methods and operations would remain significant. Although psychiatric diagnosis has been improved to some extent with the developments of the Diagnostic and Statistical Manual of Mental Disorders, Third Edition (DSM-III) (American Psychiatric Association, 1980) and the Diagnostic and Statistical Manual of Mental Disorders, Third Edition, Revised (DSM-III-R) (American Psychiatric Association, 1987), there is still a long way to go. Masserman (1979) foresees these current Linnaen-Kraepelinean diagnostic systems as being superseded by more informed multivectorial systems, and all diagnosis as ultimately based on a much fuller understanding of etiology and pathogensis than is currently the case.

Similarly, much remains to do regarding the demonstrated efficacy and specificity of the psychotherapies. Since the 1960s, when research workers crept into the psychotherapy consultation office and began to demonstrate that personality characteristics and interaction styles of the therapist transcended their theoretical orientations with respect to therapeutic impact, some of the specificity of the therapeutic claims for some psychotherapies, for at least some problems, has been in serious question, and the myth that only medical practitioners are competent to do psychotherapy has been shattered (Frank et al., 1978). Because of interests in cost containment and cost-effective services, more money may be put into evaluation research. However, this remains a difficult area of study for psychiatry.

Considerable research still needs to be conducted on assessing the effectiveness of the healing relationship and psychotherapies, as conducted by psychiatrists, other mental health professionals, and even by nonprofessionals. Self-help groups, including groups using the Alcoholics Anonymous recovery model, are very popular and should be assessed in comparison to professional interventions. Current drug-free projects for the treatment of alcoholics, substance abusers, and psychotic patients require evaluation research and may lead us to new models of understanding and treatment.

The fifth expectation, that the appropriate role of the psychiatrist would continue to be controversial, is evident in several chapters in this book. To date, no one has conducted a functional analysis of the tasks, level of knowledge, and skills necessary for the comprehensive conduct of mental health services. Such a project would permit more rational planning for the training of mental health manpower in the future, and would probably presage the development of several new mental health professions, essentially hybrids of the current ones in psychiatry, neurology, internal medicine, pediatrics, nursing, psychology, and social work. However, professional allegiances, status, economic forces, and social sanctions all retard the evolution of new administrative forms.

Another expectation, in the early and mid-1970s, was the belief that national health insurance was likely to be established (Astrachan et al, 1976; Marmor, 1976). At that time, it was unclear as to whether psychiatry would be included in national health insurance, and if so what types of services would be covered. But for the present time, at least, national health insurance appears to be a dead issue, although the question as to whether psychiatry will be covered in some nationally funded catastrophic health insurance plans remains open.

The last expectation, in the 1970s, was the prediction that a large number of social changes would produce ethical issues important to the practice of psychiatry (Toffler, 1980). These concerned changing views about sexuality, the roles of women, abortion, attitudes toward self-determination regarding death and the manner of dying, and so forth. These all remain current issues.

Fancifully, for the future we can imagine new types of adjustment reactions and identity disorders as social forms, values, and ethical issues change. If communal marriages were to occur, for example, what psychological problems might occur through the dissolution of a three- or four-way marriage? A trivorce or quadrivorce rather than divorce? If values change so that additional types of problems, formerly conceived as misfortunes, become redefined as injustices, with the victims seeking redress, how might psychiatry be affected? Such a shift in perception has already increased the number of malpractice suits against physicians. Can we anticipate changing legal relationships, for example, between children and their parents, with children divorcing parents?

The 1980s have brought predictions of even more profound and rapid changes in psychiatric practice based on several all-pervasive economic influences and trends that were just barely perceived at the beginning of the 1970s (Ginzburg 1987; Beigel, 1986; Macdonald, 1987; Talbott, 1985a, 1985b; Nadelson, 1985; Pasnau, 1987). The major forces include corporatization and cost containment. These have led to the diagnosis related group (DRG) prospective payment systems; the movement of psychiatrists to hospitals and multispecialty clinics with possibly fewer independent private office practitioners in the future; greater competition between psychiatrists and the increasing numbers of nonpsychiatric mental health professionals; increased willingness of psychiatrists to act as medical physicians; increased marketing and entrepreneurship among physicians; greater societal support for deregulation with an increase in the number of independent practitioners other than physicians (such as nurses), who can bill independently for their services; and an increase in the total number of physicians, with a predicted decrease in income per physician. Costs are also shifting the locus of care from hospitals to nonhospital alternatives, such as nursing homes or other lower cost care facilities for chronic patients.

Another current trend that may also affect psychiatry is the increasing number of worksite-based employee assistant programs (EAPs), particularly those concerned with alcohol and drug abuse. However, to date psychiatrists have been relatively uninvolved in these programs. As cost offset studies demonstrate the added value (or relative lack of added value) of psychiatrists to patient care in these and other settings, the demand for psychiatrists will correspondingly shift.

Several of the visionaries imagined the need for increased collaborative relationships between psychiatrists and nonphysician mental health professionals, through multigroup practices or through "triangle" arrangements.

Thus, social values and economic realities will continue to act as breaks or facilitators for psychiatry, in spite of advances in technology. Technological advances judged to be of major value will flourish, while other advances may lie dormant. For example, consider the speed with which magnetic resonance imaging (MRI) and computerized tomography (CT) scans have been incorporated into daily medical practice, only a few years after the basic scientific research leading to these developments was reported. In contrast, diagnostic sleep laboratories, with technology that has been well reported for more than a decade, have not developed as quickly, perhaps because of the relatively less urgent and more chronic nature of the complaints involved.

Scientific and Technological Advances

Here we can indulge in flights of fanciful imagination and attempt to envision what the application of today's basic science knowledge and unexpected new advances might portend for the practice of psychiatry and other mental health professions. At the outset, several points are in order:

Serendipity has always played a major role in treatment advances in psychiatry. For example, the clinical applications of ECT, phenothiazines, antidepressants, and lithium were all chance discoveries, unrelated to their originally intended purposes. In addition, psychiatric advances these days frequently stem from the work of nonpsychiatrists. Discoveries made in all the basic and social sciences are important. Concepts increasingly familiar in other areas of science, from information theory to physics, have affected, and will continue to percolate into, our own thinking and practice. To illustrate, Marmor (1976) pointed out how systems thinking has been influential in psychiatry over the last decade, and that viewing the individual and the family as open, rather than closed, systems has shifted attention away from isolated individuals as the appropriate unit of study and intervention (as in the case of psychoanalysis), to family and social settings as well. In partial validation of this shift, a follow-up study of University of California at Los Angeles–Neuropsychiatric Institute psychiatric residency graduates revealed that, in contrast to those who graduated during the 1960s, significantly more of the recent graduates identified marital conflicts and marital therapy as being important issues for a significant number of their patients (Yager et al., 1979), suggesting that psychiatric graduates have become more accustomed to thinking in family systems terms and are seeing patients in a different perspective.

New clinical problems will probably present a continuous challenge to the science available to us. For example, a decade ago who would have predicted the emergence of the acquired immunodeficiency syndrome (AIDS), with its major psychosocial and psychobiological implications for psychiatric research and practice?

Psychiatric visionaries have long enjoyed musing about scientific advances and their implications; many have predicted major advances in psychiatrically relevant basic and clinical sciences, based on the explosion of biological knowledge and methods in all areas of medicine (West, 1973; Masserman, 1979). One need only pick up the most recent issues of *Nature* or *Science* to witness the knowledge explosion in genetics and immunology, for example.

On a cautionary note, Leon Eisenberg (1973) suggested that, despite scientific advances, we are unlikely to eliminate the chronic psychoses and the problems that they generate. In his view, it is unlikely that genetic engineering or genetic counseling programs will seriously reduce the incidence of the psychoses. However, for the next century he predicts, "we will have reached a point at which we will structure special environments, both behavioral and biochemical, for children identified by biological indices as being at hazard for psychosis" (Eisenberg, 1973, p. 1375).

Havens (1986) expects that increased knowledge of evolution and sociobiology will lead to better understanding of pathogenesis in human psychiatric conditions, and also suggests that a nosology of human situations (not only biological and diagnostic possibilities) will lead to fresh insights into the etiology and pathogenesis of *breakdown conditions*. He envisions advances in psychotherapy, leading to a subdivision of psychotherapies by subspecialists, and improved psychological aptitude tests, enabling us to better understand and assess the available amount of "energy" an individual can devote to personal development and interpersonal relationships. New forms of psychotherapy are likely to emerge (Karasu, 1987); thus, for example, the use of videotape playback in individual and family therapy has hardly been explored.

New combinations of psychotherapy and medications, and new concepts of the use of time in psychotherapy are also likely.

Perhaps the most imaginative psychiatric futurist has been Louis Jolyon West, who, in 1973, published his speculations concerning the future of psychiatric education, a paper that slightly modified remarks originally written in 1966. Because some of West's remarks were addressed to the current decade, it is instructive to examine how accurate his prophesies were and see to what extent his predictions have come to pass. His major point was that the psychiatrist of tomorrow would be more of a synthesizer than a technical subspecialist, needing to master a broad scientific vocabulary. His thoughts are consistent with Buckminster Fuller's view that postindustrial man will be a generalist rather than a specialist, and that he will depend on machines for subspecialization (Fuller, 1972). However, as is evident from the debate earlier in this volume, subspecialization in psychiatry is still on the ascendance, and it is likely to continue so at least for the near future.

West (1973) predicted the increasing importance of mathematical modeling in psychiatric research, including models based the branch of mathematics known as topology. Indeed, an article in *Scientific American,* entitled "Catastrophe Theory," described applications of topology to understanding decision making in highly uncertain situations and in anorexia nervosa (Zeeman, 1976).

West also mentioned advances in psychophysics, three-dimensional wave models, and cybernetics; that consciousness would reemerge as an area of interest; that autonomic profiles and possibly enzyme-screening batteries may impact on practice. In research, these areas were already under very active investigation, as in the work of Pribram on holographic models of the mind and of Sperry and others on localization of brain (if not mind) function. Electronics, data processing, cultural anthropology, and sociology were all cited by West as areas likely to provide advances. He further stated that "in ten years . . . every young psychiatrist will understand how to employ computerized EEG's" (West, 1973, p. 528).

Although it is now 15 years after the publication of West's paper, the basic advances he mentioned have not filtered very far into clinical practice. While his prediction that the psychiatrist of tomorrow would be more of a neuroscientist than a psychotherapist may be coming to pass, the shift so far has not been dramatic. But we are still evolving in this direction (Detre, 1987), and psychiatrists do seem to be relatively more occupied with the care of the seriously mentally ill than they were two decades ago, in line with West's prediction.

There is one lesson to be gleaned from this historical perspective on West's paper: given the economics of health care, new advances will translate into clinical practice only after they have been shown to have true therapeutic worth. Ths was the case with lithium carbonate, and the clinical values of other putative advances, such as the dexamethasone suppression test (American Psychiatric Association Task Force on Laboratory Tests in Psychiatry, 1987), various neuroendocrine challenge tests, and the monitoring of some drug blood values, are still in question.

Additional predictions about the future of psychiatry can be made by extending current technologies and by imagining extensions of basic research to psychiatric practice.

Molecular genetics is exploding, and it is exciting to contemplate exactly what clinical advances for psychiatry will follow complete mapping of the human genome. Likewise, DNA splicing could ultimately provide unimagined accomplishments.

Antisera for specific brain receptors and other advances in immunology may lead to more precise cerebral localization studies. Immunological discoveries could lead to discrete molecular interventions targeted at specific brain regions, far more sophisticated than today's shotgun approach with drugs that affect a wide array of brain systems and other organs. Antigens may provide markers for specific types of susceptibility, as for example, in certain species of pigs, the H blood antigen has been shown to predict stress susceptibility. We may be able to develop vaccines against alcoholism, smoking, drug abuse, and other behavioral conditions.

Brain transplants, hardly believed possible decades ago, have already been shown to be in part workable in animals and in the treatment of Parkinson's disease in humans. Currently under investigation are new models of nerve action based on local circuits, wave forms of cortical event-related potentials, and immunological determinants of neural organization. We require new ways of thinking about the organization of nerve nets, and questions regarding subtle sensing systems in man demand study: do we have sensors that respond to magnetic, electrical, atmospheric, gravitational, high and low frequency vibration, or pheromone-like cues? Advances in biophysics may lead to new information regarding the organization of information and consciousness. New methods of brain imaging, the next generations of PET and MRI scanners, promise much better understanding of brain structure and function.

Discoveries are awaited in chronobiology, and enzymology and pharmacology are still young fields. We can anticipate better understandings of temperament and cognitive style, through advances in genetic and developmental psychobiology. Such advances will also reveal more about the innate structures of grammar, language, and thought, and about the nature of disturbances in those systems.

How will advances in artificial intelligence influence psychiatric practice? Currently, computer terminals are envisioned in every physician's office to assist in diagnosis, workup, and treatment, with expert systems asking questions and offering suggestions at every stage (Barnett et al., 1987; Shortliffe, 1987). Currently, microcomputers are capable of administering a large number of psychological tests and structured psychiatric interviews (Williams and Johnson, 1979; Maxmen, 1976). Expert-system computer programs have already demonstrated their practical clinical utility as therapeutic adjuncts in short-term psychotherapy for situational crises and adjustment problems (Gould, 1986). Ultimately, whole families may be assessed with the help of computers using psychological, psychophysiological, and biological instrumentation, providing treatment strategies and prognostic statements based on family members' temperaments, cognitive styles, communication patterns, and types of interactional difficulties.

Computer-assisted consultation, particularly regarding psychopharmacological information and other data-based knowledge, should shortly be available in all offices and emergency rooms. Toffler (1980) discusses OLIVER, an On-Line Interactive Vicarious Expediter and Responder, a personal computer that may hold all the information we ever need, know our values, and be able to help us make decisions. One could imagine that such computers could be used to provide patients instant access to advice and counseling and could contain individually designed optimal therapeutic characteristics akin to Jiminy Cricket or HAL, the computer in "2001: A Space Odyssey."

Shaping our Futures

A primary reason for studying the future is to influence it. Given the diversity of opinions about the definition of psychiatry, the proper role of the psychiatrist, and the multiple value-laden social and scientific considerations that enter these opinions, it is not surprising that psychiatric prophets and policy makers have offered a wide range of views as to how psychiatry should organize and orient itself for the future.

Talbott (1985a, 1985b) cautions that psychiatry should assure, first and foremost, that the large numbers of patients in our society who have acute and chronic mental illnesses will be properly cared for by psychiatrists, and not abandoned by them. He admonishes psychiatry to improve the delivery systems for psychiatric care so that, even with limited funding, systems are established in which the available money follows the patients. We should abandon systems that lose interest once the patient is discharged from their narrow fields of responsibility and institute over-arching systems, in which the patient, perhaps through the use of vouchers, can be followed continuously from hospital to outpatient care setting. MacDonald, recently administrator of the Alcohol, Drug Abuse, and Mental Health Administration, also warns psychiatrists to attend to many of the current economic and public care issues, lest they become irrelevant and ignored by corporations and federal funding agencies alike (Macdonald, 1987). He believes that psychiatrists must continue to involve themselves in public psychiatry via state hospitals, the employee assistance program movement, nursing homes, and the care of the chronically mentally ill, dual-diagnosis, substance-abusing patients and psychiatric patients with medical problems.

What will be the role of psychiatrists vis-à-vis other health professionals? Pardes (1979), citing data to show that primary care physicians often don't recognize or adequately treat psychiatric problems, states that psychiatrists have the unique capabilities and responsibilities to diagnose and consult on patients with psychiatric disorders, and to treat them as well. However, with regard to treatment, Pardes sees psychiatrists working in collaboration with other mental health professionals, triaging patients to them for care as appropriate. Neill and Ludwig (1980, p. 39), asking "whither psychotherapy in psychiatry?" believe that psychiatrists may do "medically indicated" psychotherapy, which would include extended physical-neurological assessments and combined psychotherapy-psychopharmacology management. Other areas would depend on demonstrated cost effectiveness and technical specificity. In their view, psychiatrists will not be able to simply do mystical, existential, and affectual psychotherapy within the confines and constraints of the prospective payment system.

In one of the most clearly delineated visions of future psychiatry, Detre (1987) suggests that tomorrow's psychiatrist will be a clinical neuroscientist. His views suggest that preparation for a psychiatric career should include adequate exposure to medicine, neurology, psychiatry, and pharmacology and that it should also include teaching in clinical neuropsychology, electrophysiology, and imaging. Psychiatric residents would be taught critical problem-solving skills to prepare them for the explosion of knowledge and to allow them to be sophisticated consumers of technical science. They should also be psychosocially competent, to avoid being too biologically focused (although in his view the interactive and interpersonal skills necessary for the psychiatrist are not the exclusive domain of psychiatry, but belong to all of medicine). Detre also envisions this clinical neuroscientist as one who can practice informed consent, that is, one who can educate and interact with patients on the costs and benefits of the various treatments available and help them decide, in an informed way based on data rather than on myth, what treatment options are available to them.

In this regard, Heinz Lehmann (1986), a highly regarded psychopharmacology researcher, provides some useful cautionary comments. He sees himself not as a pessimist, but as a realist who envisions psychiatry in competition with both other physicians and nonphysician mental health practitioners. In his view, all acute psychiatric problems should be the domain of the psychiatrist, who, after an assessment and emergency or urgent treatment, would either continue to treat the patients if indicated or turn their care over to colleagues. To remain clinically relevant in the marketplace, psychiatrists will have to be highly available for emergency consultations and able to make useful interventions quickly.

However, in the face of the neuroscience explosion, Lehmann (1986, p. 367) asks, "Is psychiatry in the process of selling its birthright for a mess of technological hardware, molecular biology and highly reliable diagnostic algorithms of questionable validity? Have we mortgaged psychiatry's future to technological potential?" His response, and mine, is that tomorrow's psychiatrists must be extremely well informed about and competent in handling the technology, but the technology has to be in the service of the physician, and the physician has to be in the service of the patient, not the other way around.

Summary

Attempts to predict the future of psychiatry from what has preceded may seem foolhardy, yet certain trends emerge. Given respect for the inertia of social and economic systems, we can venture some educated guesses.

In spite of the homogenizing effects on American culture of the mass media, we can anticipate still greater complexity, differentiation, and diversity in American lifestyles, ethnic groups, and social classes. The practice patterns of various mental health professionals will further differentiate, to best cater to the needs of these population subgroups, each with its own values, belief systems, health care practices, and health service utilization patterns.

We can anticipate an increased bureaucratization of psychiatric practice. Federal government regulations, corporatization, and the burgeoning of quasiregulatory agencies contribute to this trend.

Funding for psychiatric care is not likely to increase because of cost containment efforts. However, the new emergence of active lobbying groups, organized by families of the mentally ill, may result in increased money for chronic care services and research in certain localized areas.

The percentage of the population seeking mental health services will increase (as it did between 1955, when it was one percent, and 1980, when it was six percent). In spite of the increasing numbers of nonphysician mental health professionals, as well as psychiatrists, the prevalence of emotional disorders in the population is so high that, if funds were available, all trained professionals would be busy. Collaborative rather than competitive attitudes among the health and mental health professions are likely to be in everyone's best interests, when attempting to increase funding for these disorders.

Thousands of papers and a few new ideas will continue to tumble out of the laboratories in dozens of biological and social science disciplines. They will generate much enthusiasm, new hypotheses and paradigms, and additional research. Many ideas and findings will fall by the wayside, but some will stand the test of time and ultimately be translated into practical beneficial therapies.

Increasing specificity in psychiatric diagnosis will be based on greater scientific understanding of etiology and pathogenesis. We can anticipate new complexity and substantial changes in the psychiatric workup, so that comprehensive diagnosis will less frequently be based on the history and mental status examination alone. In this fashion, psychiatry will follow internal medicine and other medical specialties, which have witnessed the increased use of laboratory procedures for accurate assessment.

Psychotherapies of various types will continue to proliferate with enormous speed, and these will continue to have half lives of about two to five years. Any therapy that lasts more than one generation (one that outlives its originator) and that develops a loyal group of adherents who publish a journal persisting for more than a decade will deserve to be written up in subsequent editions of the Comprehensive Textbook of Psychiatry (Kaplan and Sadock, 1985).

Insurance companies will continue to restrict reimbursement. They will attempt to pay only for those biological and therapeutic strategies that are demonstrated to be more potent than placebo or that deliver measurable improvements in the quality of life in chronic conditions.

With all of these developments, we can anticipate further sub-specialization within psychiatry. And finally, primitive fears to the contrary, it is likely that current psychiatric graduates who show reasonable intelligence, competence, commitment to continuing education, resourcefulness, and motivation will not want for work.

Coping Methods

Methods for coping with the rapid changes buffeting psychiatry are needed by the profession and by individual psychiatrists. In my view, the profession will best survive if it fosters allegiance to patient care, to function rather than to form, and to tasks rather than to professional identity boundaries. Psychiatry must design service strategies that simultaneously take excellent care of patients, acknowledge and work along with other health and mental health professionals, and respect all concerned.

Research into the tasks of psychiatric health care delivery might point to new functional organization of the professions. Exactly what do psychiatrists need to know to make their clinical decisions? To what extent do others or can others have the training to allow them to undertake at least some of those activities in a competent fashion? The same questions are currently being asked regarding the role and training of nurse practitioners and physicians assistants in internal medicine, pediatrics, and anesthesia; optometrists vis-à-vis ophthalmalogists; dentists vis-à-vis oral surgeons; podiatrists vis-à-vis orthopedists; and so forth.

The profession must continue to educate the public and to lobby at all governmental levels for the inclusion of psychiatric benefits in public and private insurance plans. How effectively are we lobbying and organizing those legislators who, by virtue of personal experiences with the needs of relatives and significant others for psychiatric services, might constitute the most determined and outspoken to promote mental health-oriented legislation? The American Psychiatric Association should also continue its organized activities in future-oriented, long-term planning.

How can individuals cope? Good copers demonstrate flexibility, rationality, awareness of social influences, and the capacity to engage in rehearsals and trial actions in advance of stress. To start, realism suggests that some forms of individual practice, as well as some forms of therapy, will become progressively obsolete. They will be replaced by other forms of more clearly demonstrable cost-effective care.

Recognizing the explosion of knowledge, most authorities acknowledge that three or four years of training is insufficient. Active methods of learning are much more powerful than passive methods, and, given the pressure for time, nothing should be included in the curriculum unless it can be justified in terms of future use. Some futuristic methods are applicable to residency training, as, for example, interactive games are frequently more instructive than lectures or seminars. Thus, residents learning administration could be challenged to design an ideal impatient service, clinic, or alternative service system, into which various constraints are injected. To learn forensic psychiatry residents could participate in mock court with law students. Other issues of particular pertinence to residency training are discussed by Kay and Tasman in Chapter 7.

Increasing numbers of residency graduates are taking fellowships, staying on medical school faculties, attending professional meetings and conferences, requesting consultations from psychiatric subspecialists, and engaging in many other continuing-education activities. Telephone, videophone, and computer-mediated consultation services should all be used to keep current and to upgrade one's level of practice. Part-time post graduate continuing education courses through university extension divisions and refresher clerkships, that include didactic and clinical experiences, may be of particular benefit.

Group practices may be more adaptive than solo practices, and a variety of interesting group practice arrangements have been described among psychiatrists, psychiatrists in collaboration with other mental health professionals, psychiatrists in collaboration with other medical specialists, and around certain specialty problems. Such group practices might facilitate lifelong learning, with group members taking time off for continuing education, which could include longer sabbaticals for in-residence refresher clerkships.

We are moving from what Margaret Mead (1970) has called a postfigurative culture, where the young learn from the old, through a cofigurative culture, where children and adults learn mainly from their peers, to prefigurative educational cultures, where the old learn from the young. We will always have a lot to learn, and there will be no room for complacency. One thing can be predicted with certainty: the future of psychiatry will not be boring!

References

American Medical Association Council on Long Range Planning and Development: The future of medicine: a scenario analysis. JAMA 1987; 250:80–85

American Psychiatric Association: Diagnostic and Statistical Manual of Mental Disorders, Third Edition. Washington, DC, American Psychiatric Association, 1980

American Psychiatric Association: Diagnostic and Statistical Manual of Mental Disorders, Third Edition, Revised. Washington, DC, American Psychiatric Association, 1987

American Psychiatric Association Task Force on Laboratory Tests in Psychiatry: The dexamethasone suppression test: an overview of its current status in psychiatry. Am J Psychiatry 1987; 144:1253–1262

Astrachan BM, Levinson DJ, Adler DA: The impact of national health insurance on the tasks and practice of psychiatry. Arch Gen Psychiatry 1976; 33: 785–794

Barnett GO, Cimino JJ, Hupp JA, et al: DXplain: an evolving diagnostic decision support system. JAMA 1987; 258:67–74

Beigel A: Planning psychiatry's future. Hosp Community Psychiatry 1986; 37:551–554

Bell D (ed): Toward the Year 2000: Work in Progress. New York, Beacon Press, 1968, pp 1–20, 378–381

Calder N: 1984 and Beyond. New York, Viking Press, 1984, pp 7–103

Cetron M, O'Toole T: Encounters with the Future. New York, McGraw Hill, 1982

Clare A: Chapter 2, in *Psychiatrists on Psychiatry*. Edited by Shepherd M. London, Cambridge University Press, 1982

Clarke AC: Technology and the future, in Report on Planet Three. Edited by Clarke AC. New York, Signet Publishers, 1972, pp 129–141

Detre T: The future of psychiatry. Am J Psychiatry 1987; 144:621–625

Eisenberg L: The future of psychiatry. Lancet 1973; 2:1371–1375

Frank J, Hoehn–Saric R, Imber S, et al: Effective Ingredients of Successful Psychotherapy. New York, Brunner/Mazel, 1978

Freedman A: Creating the future. Am J Psychiatry 1974; 131:749–754

Freedman DX: Science in the service of the ill. Am J Psychiatry 1982; 139:1087–1095

Fuller RB: Technology and the human environment, in The Futurists. Edited by Toffler A. New York, Random House, 1972, pp 298–306

Ginzburg E: Psychiatry before the year 2000: the long view. Hosp Community Psychiatry 1987; 38:725–728

Gordon TJ: The current methods of future research, in The Futurists. Edited by Toffler A. New York, Random House, 1972, pp 164–189

Gordon WJJ: Synectics: The Development of Creative Capacities. New York, Collier, 1961

Gould RL: The therapeutic learning program: a computer assisted short term treatment program. Computers in Psychiatry/Psychology 1986; 8:7–12

Harris M: America Now: The Anthropology of a Changing Culture. New York, Simon & Schuster, 1981

Havens LL: Why the future belongs to psychiatry. Psychother Psychosom 1986; 45:14–22

Helmer O: Prospects of technological progress, in The Futurists. Edited by Toffler A. New York, Random House, 1972, pp 151–159

Institute for Alternative Futures, Future Mental Health Services Project: Scenarios for the Future of Mental Health Services. Alexandria, VA, Institute for Alternative Futures, 1985

Jungk R: Evolution and revolution in the west, in The Futurists. Edited by Toffler A. New York, Random House, 1972, pp 73–84

Kahn H, Weiner AJ: The next thirty–three years: a framework for speculation, in Toward the Year 2000. Edited by Bell D. New York, Beacon Books, 1969, pp 73–100

Kahn H, Brown W, Martel L, et al: The Next 200 Years. New York, William Morrow, 1976, 1–25, 181–207

Kaplan HI, Sadock BJ (eds): Comprehensive Textbook of Psychiatry IV, Fourth edition. Baltimore, Williams & Wilkins, 1985

Karasu TB: The psychotherapy of the future. Psychosomatics 1987; 28:380–384

Kuhn TS: The Structure of Scientific Revolutions. Chicago, University of Chicago Press, 1962

Langsley DG: Today's teachers and tomorrow's psychiatrists. Am J Psychiatry 1981; 138:1013–1016

Lehmann HE: The future of psychiatry: progress, mutation—or self-destruct? Can J Psychiatry 1986; 31:362–36

Macdonald DI: Future psychiatric services. Paper presented at Annual Meeting of American Psychiatric Association, Chicago, IL, May 1987

Majno C, Sanchez GC, Scully RE: Bicentennial Clinical Pathological Conference: syphillis, diarrhea and death in the 1820's. N Engl J Med 1976; 295:1592–1600

Marmor J: Psychiatry 1976—the continuing revolution. Am J Psychiatry 1976; 133:739–745

Masserman JH: The future of psychiatry as a scientific and humanitarian discipline in a changing world. Am J Psychiatry 1979; 136:1013–1019

Maxmen JS: The Post-Physician Era: Medicine in the 21st century. New York, John Wiley & Sons, 1976

Maxmen JS: Telecommunications in psychiatry. Am J Psychiatry 1978; 32:450–456

Mead M: The future: prefigurative cultures and unknown children, Culture and Commitment. Edited by Mead M. New York, Doubleday, 1970, pp 27–50

Nadelson CC: Health care direction: who cares for patients? Am J Psychiatry 1986; 143:949–955

Naisbitt J: Megatrends: Ten New Directions Transforming Our Lives. New York, Warner Books, 1984, pp xxii–xxxii

Naisbitt J, the Naisbitt Group: The Year Ahead. 1986: Ten Powerful Trends Shaping Your Future. New York, Warner Books, 1985

Neill JR, Ludwig AM: Psychiatry and psychotherapy: past and future. Am J Psychother 1980; 34:39–50

Pardes H: Future needs for psychiatrists and other mental health personnel. Arch Gen Psychiatry 1979; 36:1401–1408

Pasnau RO: Psychiatry in medicine: medicine in psychiatry. Am J Psychiatry 1987; 144:975–980

Renfro WL: Future histories: a new approach to scenarios. The Futurists 1987; 21:38–41

Shortliffe EH: Computer programs to support clinical decision making. JAMA 1987; 258:61–66

Strauss G, Yager J, Strauss G: The cutting edge in psychiatry. Am J Psychiatry 1984; 141:38–43

Talbott JA: Our patients' future in a changing world: the imperative for psychiatric involvement in public policy. Am J Psychiatry 1985a; 142:1003–1008

Talbott JA: The fate of the public psychiatric system. Hosp Community Psychiatry 1985b; 36:46–50

Tarjan G: American psychiatry: a dynamic mosaic. Am J Psychiatry 1984; 141:923–927

Toffler A (ed): Future Shock. New York, Random House, 1970

Toffler A (ed): The Futurists. New York, Random House, 1973, pp 3–10, 96–130

Toffler A: The psychology of the future, in Learning for Tomorrow: the Role of the Future in Education. Edited by Toffler A. New York, Vintage Press, 1974, pp 3–19

Toffler A: The Third Wave. New York, William Morrow, 1980

Toffler A: Previews and Premises. New York, William Morrow, 1983

Torrey FE: The Death of Psychiatry. New York, Penguin Books, 1974

Waskow AI: (1972). Towards a democratic futurism, in The Futurists. Edited by Toffler A. New York, Random House, 1972, pp 85–95

West LJ: The future of psychiatric education. Am J Psychiatry 1973; 130:521–528

Williams TA, Johnson JF (eds): Mental Health in the 21st Century. Lexington Books, D.C. Heath and Co., 1979

Yager J, Pasnau RO, Lipschultz S: Professional characteristics of psychiatric residents trained at the UCLA Neuropsychiatric Institute 1956–1975. Journal of Psychiatric Education 1979; 3:72–85

Zeeman EC: Catastrophe theory. Scientific American 1976; 234:65–83